Props for *Vegan Soul Kitchen:*
Fresh, Healthy, and Creative African American Cuisine

"Bryant Terry's warm hearted, soulful dishes shout out to you and me with crackling, lip-smacking goodness. His fresh and sassy way at the stove puts meat on the bones of the very plants that are sure to sustain us for generations to come. "
   —Peter Berley, author of *The Flexitarian Table*

"Bryant has written a very creative, original, and musical cookbook. I look forward to trying out a bunch of these appetizing recipes. As a teacher, seeing a graduate of the Natural Gourmet Institute succeed so beautifully warms my heart."
   —Annemarie Colbin, Ph.D., founder, The Natural Gourmet
      Institute for Health and Culinary Arts, author of
      The Whole-Food Guide to Strong Bones

"Bryant Terry transforms age-old black culinary traditions into what soul food ought to be—food that sustain our bodies, our earth, our sense of community, and our desire for the delicious. For the naysayers who resist the audacity of okra or the soft power of tofu, *Vegan Soul Kitchen* is the new manifesto that cries out, Yes We Can give up meat and enjoy gastronomic nirvana."
   —Robin D. G. Kelley, author of
      Freedom Dreams: The Black Radical Imagination

"Anyone with soul and good taste will love Bryant's 'Afro-Diasporic' recipes. They're downright delicious and satisfying. By mixing together the freshest beats with local, sustainable ingredients and healthful cooking techniques, Bryant brings to life the festive culture of celebration that comes from eating this way."
   —Ani Phyo, author of *Ani's Raw Food Kitchen* and
      Ani's Raw Food Desserts

"That boy can cook!"
—Ann Peebles, Singer and Songwriter (and Bryant's Aunt)

"Don't let the 'Vegan' in the title fool you. With food, music, and a zero waste way with watermelon that yields 6 recipes, Bryant Terry's *Vegan Soul Kitchen* is not just for vegans. Innovative and taste-full recipes like Sweet Cornmeal Coconut Drop Biscuits, and Baked BBQ Black Eyed Peas, make it a book for anyone who wants to eat well."
—Jessica B. Harris, professor, food historian, lecturer,
    and author of ten cookbooks

"As the chef and owner of Farmer Brown Restaurant, I know first-hand the challenges of bringing soul food to people who haven't tried it. If you're new to this cuisine, Bryant Terry's recipes will open your world; if you're looking for a twist, prepare to be amazed. All I can say is WOW! Thank you Bryant."
—Jay Foster, Farmer Brown Restaurant

"A pioneer of the East Coast food justice movement, now hailing from the West Coast home of progressive food politics—where the Black Panther Party's Free Breakfast for Children program made nutrition a key ingredient of social transformation and where Alice Waters started an organic revolution—who else but Chef Bryant Terry could have brought us the finger-licking, ethical eats in *Vegan Soul Kitchen*. At a moment when food can harm as well as heal, he has ingeniously re-imagined soul food by going back to the roots *and* back to the land. Recipes paired with vintage R&B, praise songs and poetry remind us that African diasporic cuisine has always been food for living and a total sensory experience."
—Alondra Nelson, Yale University, author of *Body and Soul:*
    The Black Panther Party and the Politics of Race and Health

VEGAN SOUL KITCHEN

VEGAN
SOUL
KITCHEN BRYANT TERRY

**FRESH, HEALTHY, AND CREATIVE
AFRICAN AMERICAN CUISINE**

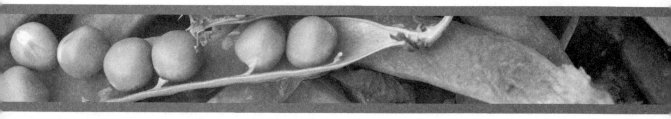

Da Capo

∞

LIFE
LONG

A Member of the Perseus Books Group

Song © 2009 Donald Bryant
Foreword © 2009 Myra Kornfeld
Poem © 2009 Michael Molina
Food Styling by Erin Quon: www.erinquon.com
Photographs by Sara Remington, Keba Konte, and
    Brittany M. Powell

Designed by Trish Wilkinson
Set in 11.5 point Minion

Library of Congress Cataloging-in-Publication Data

Terry, Bryant, 1974–
    Vegan Soul kitchen : fresh, healthy, and creative African American cuisine / Bryant Terry. — 1st Da Capo Press ed.
        p.   cm.
    ISBN 978-0-7382-1228-9 (alk. paper)
    1. Vegan cookery. 2. African American cookery. 3. Cookery, American—Southern style. I. Title.
TX837.T434 2009
641.5'636—dc22   2008046945

First Da Capo Press edition 2009
ISBN: 978-0-7382-1228-9

Published by Da Capo Press
A Member of the Perseus Books Group
www.dacapopress.com

Da Capo Press books are available at special discounts for bulk purchases in the United States by corporations, institutions, and other organizations. For more information, please contact the Special Markets Department at the Perseus Books Group, 2300 Chestnut Street, Suite 200, Philadelphia, PA 19103, or call (800) 810-4145, extension 5000, or e-mail special.markets@perseusbooks.com.

In memory of my grandparents
Margie and Edward Bryant
&
Rosa Lee and Andrew Johnson Terry I

vsk

CONTENTS

MIX PLATES: SALADS. SLAWS. DRESSINGS.   57

LIQUID LESSONS: SOUPS. STEWS. POT LIKKER.   75

Stocks and Broths

Soups

Stews

BLESSING
by Donald Bryant

Thankful

Don Bryant

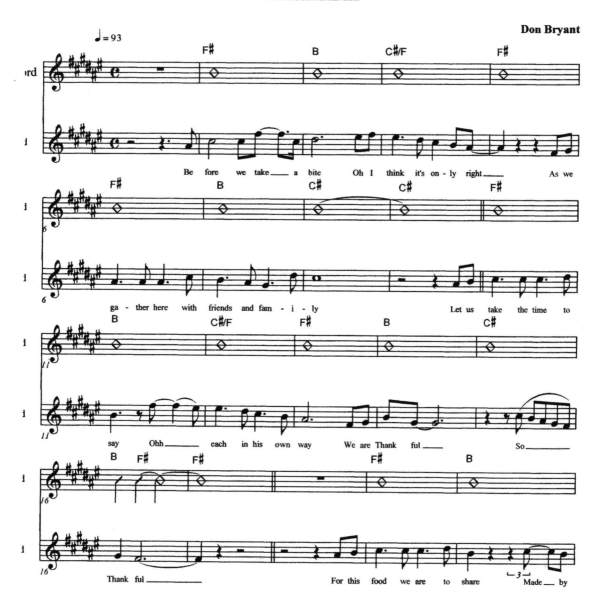

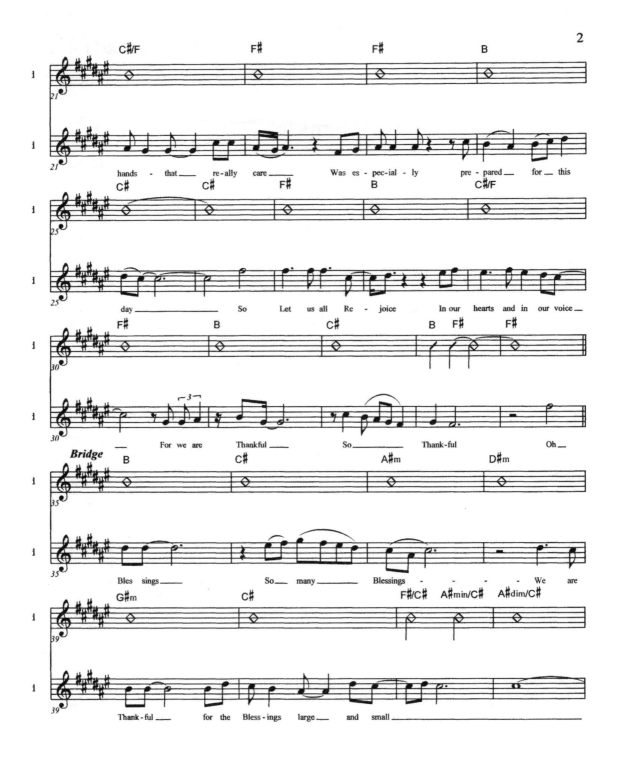

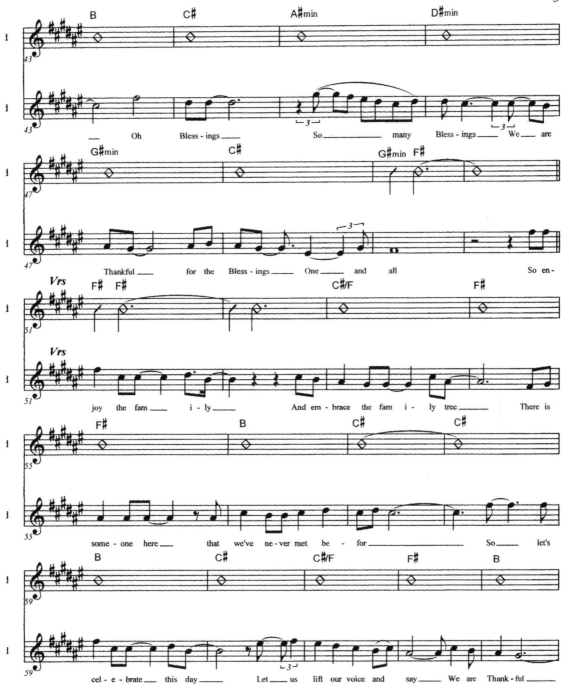

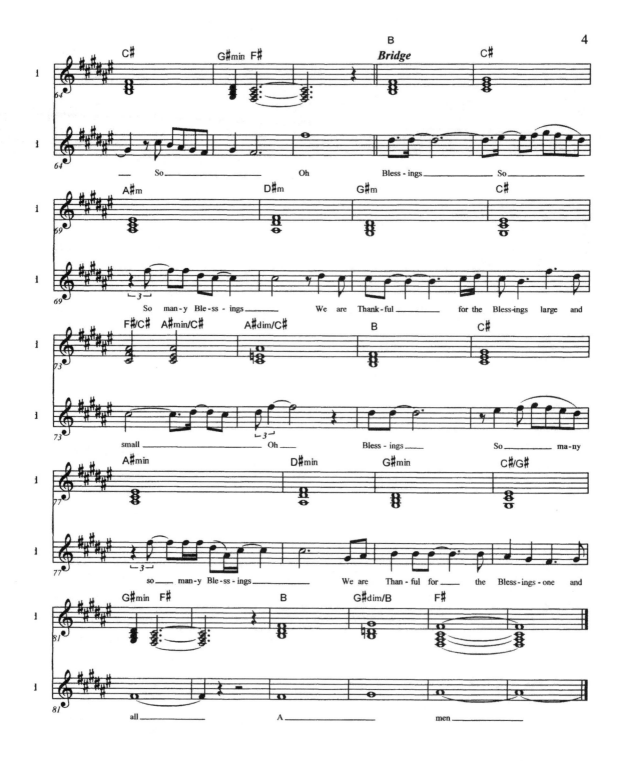

FOREWORD
by Myra Kornfeld

I like real food, and I'm glad that Bryant Terry does, too. As he says, *Vegan Soul Kitchen* is a real food cookbook for anyone with soul who likes tasty eats.

Bryant has done an accomplished job of drawing on mostly Southern and African traditions in a creative way, retaining cultural complexity while making vegan food with a distinctive soul food twist to it. He does not sacrifice flavor for health, yet the dishes are naturally healthy. You won't find textured vegetable protein, corn syrup, genetically modified fats, processed flours, or postindustrial packaged foods in these recipes. What you will find is good-quality traditional fats, and enough in each recipe to make the dish tasty. Bryant is not afraid to use the long-vilified coconut oil, an extraordinarily healthy and delicious oil that only in the last decade has been getting attention for its wonderful properties. He recommends using good-quality sea salt in place of refined table salt, and enough of it to draw the constituent flavors in a dish together. He judiciously uses high-quality sweeteners such as agave, unbleached white flour, canned tomatoes, and coconut milk. Seitan, tempeh, and agar may be unfamiliar if you are not conversant with vegan staples, but adding them to your food vocabulary expands your repertoire deliciously. The major emphasis, however, is on local and seasonal produce. When a recipe is as simple as a chilled tomato soup topped with a salsa, the tomatoes had better be in season. We are fortunate that a growing movement of local farming has yielded excellent food choices, from heirloom produce to wonderful animal products, raised in traditional humane ways.

There are no politics of veganism in this book. Bryant rightly points out that one's food journey is a personal odyssey, one that changes and alters throughout a lifetime. I wrote my first book, *The Voluptuous Vegan*, after years of working in a vegan restaurant. Nowadays I find myself frequently cooking real food for people with all different eating preferences and needs, including vegans, vegetarians, and omnivores. I love flavorful food and am adamant that vegan food should meet a high standard for flavor. I'm not one to eat something just because it is good for me, and I'm glad to say that neither is Bryant.

Bryant has examined his Memphis roots, mixed them with his lifetime of experience, and created these new, innovative, healthy versions of his favorite dishes.

Similarly, he encourages you to "remix" these recipes, modify them as best fits your personal food odyssey, play, create, and get expansive with these dishes. The soundtracks suggested for each dish add another level of creativity and spice. When you're in the kitchen you are the DJ at your own party. Make sure you've put a lot of soul in your mix.

Foreword: Myra Kornfeld

I know you got soul, if you didn't you wouldn't be in here.
—Bobby Byrd, "I Know You Got Soul"

I didn't see the type of things I wanted to see so I did it myself.
—Melvin Van Peebles, *How to Eat Your*
Watermelon in White Company (and Enjoy It)

The seed for *Vegan Soul Kitchen* was sown on Planet Brooklyn back in 2003. That spring I was asked to submit a recipe for a new book—*Recipes from America's Small Farms: Fresh Ideas for the Season's Bounty*—that celebrated the growth of the Community Supported Agriculture (CSA) movement in America. Lori Stein, the editor, was harvesting recipes from chefs, farmers, and CSA members across the country. She wanted easy-to-prepare dishes made from seasonal ingredients, mostly obtained from a typical farm box that came from a CSA. I told her that I wanted my first published recipe to have the "texture of autobiography." She liked the sound of that. So for a few days after our conversation I dug deep to come up with a dish that had some Memphis Soul

(my past) mixed with Brooklyn Boom-Bap (my present) finished off with a squeeze of Oakland Free-Range Funk (my soon-to-be future).

I decided to start with collard greens. In my mind, they were the quintessential staple of African American cooking. Paw Paw, my paternal grandfather, had at least half a dozen rows of them planted in his backyard garden that I would play in as a child. Meltingly tender collards served in an enormous steel pot made more appearances on my family's holiday tables than any other vegetable. And whenever the subject of "Soul Food" came up those blue-green cousins of kale would inevitably be mentioned within the first few sentences of the conversation. I figured that more than any other food, collards would serve as the consummate ambassador for what I imagined as my people's cuisine.

I was used to eating collards that had been simmered over low heat for an extended period of time, at least two hours, until they were a dull-green-bordering-on-brown color. While I tremendously enjoyed the rich flavor of greens (and the accompanying gravy or "pot likker") prepared this way, I was always turned off by their appearance. So I decided that I would blanch mine in salted boiling water, drain them, shock them in ice water to stop the cooking and set their color, then quickly sauté them with extra-virgin olive oil, minced garlic, and a dusting of coarse sea salt. It was an extreme departure from the way I saw greens cooked while I was growing up, but I wanted mine to appear bright, bold, and sexy!

The presentation needed to be modern and chic, too. I figured I would put some of my culinary education to use (I was at the Natural Gourmet Institute for Health and Culinary Arts at the time) and cut them into a chiffonade by removing the spines, stacking several leaves, rolling them into a tight cylinder, and slicing the leaves on a diagonal into elegant, thin strips.

The defining ingredients, the ones that would perplex people when they heard the name of this dish, would be Thompson raisins and freshly squeezed orange juice. The plump raisins would provide naturally sweet bursts of flavor. And the orange

juice's subtle tanginess would pull everything together. More than intensifying the taste of this sweet-leaning variation of a vegetable traditionally eaten savory, however, the raisins and orange juice served as a metaphor for the direction that I envisioned African American cuisine heading in the twenty-first century—more creative, cutting-edge, and refreshing.

This book could have easily been called *Citrus Collards with Raisins: Recipes as Autobiography*. As you will soon discover, *Vegan Soul Kitchen* is a succulent gumbo filled with accounts of my life, recipes, and historical notes on what I broadly define as Afro-Diasporic cuisine. Similar to my process for creating the above dish, I ruminated on my family's history and my life's trajectory to determine what recipes I would develop.

I peppered these pages with reinterpretations of popular dishes that I have eaten from countries in Africa and the Caribbean. But African American and Southern dishes enjoyed while growing up in Memphis, living in New Orleans, and traveling throughout the South inspired the bulk of these recipes. While most of them use staples associated with African American and Southern cooking, a lot of the dishes may be unfamiliar to readers . . . I mean this is a vegan cookbook.

I do realize that veganism—the avoidance of meat, poultry, seafood, eggs, dairy products, and honey—is antithetical to the way that African American and Southern cooking has been constructed in the popular imagination over the past four decades. For most people, African American and Southern cooking is synonymous with meals organized around fatty meats with overcooked vegetables and fruits playing a minor supporting role. But when we take a step back and remember that—before the widespread industrialization of food in this country—African Americans living in the South included lots of fresh, nutrient-dense leafy greens, tubers, and fruits in their everyday diets, what I am introducing here is not that much of a stretch.

For me the focus of this book is about the creative use of nutrient-dense vegetables, fresh fruits, nuts, seeds, whole grains, and legumes to make some bangin' dishes. But I do think it is important to celebrate the fact that there is this type of book available for people who enjoy African American and Southern cuisine. While I would never argue that veganism is a panacea, more and more studies are proving that properly executed vegan diets are highly beneficial for cleansing and detoxing as well as lowering the risk for and ameliorating some chronic illnesses. In fact, a study confirmed that a low-fat vegan diet might be more effective at managing type-2 diabetes than the diet recommended by the American Diabetic Association.[1] Even Oprah Winfrey went on a twenty-one-day vegan diet in June 2008 for a tune-up.[2]

I maintained a vegan diet for several years in college. After gorging myself on McDonald's, Burger King, Wendy's, and a lot of other junk foods in high school, my body was telling me to take a break from meat and dairy. Soon after I'd made that dietary shift, I learned a lot about the spiritual, moral, ethical, and environmental benefits of veganism and continued to develop compassion toward all living beings, most importantly myself. And physically, I felt exhilarated and light sustaining a vegan diet. Trusting Mother Nature's wisdom, I let the season's bounty dictate my everyday meals. In spring and summer that meant light, simple dishes mostly prepared at home—raw salads and fresh fruits; vegetables that had been steamed or cooked in very little fat; nuts and seeds; whole grains; and tempeh cooked without much fuss. In the fall and winter, I enjoyed warming

1. Caroline Wilbert, "Vegan Diet Good for Type 2 Diabetes," *CBS News* (October 1, 2008). Available online at: http://www.cbsnews.com/stories/2008/10/02/health/webmd/main4495043.shtml?source =search_story.

2. Oprah Winfrey, "The 21-Day Cleanse," *Oprah's Blog*, Week One: Sunday. Accessed online October 12, 2008, at http://www.oprah.com/article/food/healthyeating/20080520_orig_cleanse_blog1.

soups and stews; I roasted vegetables often; and I ate more heavy, grounding foods to keep me warm.

I know my story and recipes will speak to vegans, but it is also important for me to reach those whose eating habits don't fall neatly into one dietary construct or another but who are open to exploring the benefits of veganism and have a hunch that it doesn't mean being hemmed in by a few ingredients or cooking styles. In the end, I hope to inspire everyone to consider the most important lesson that I have learned throughout my journey with food: pay close attention and listen to my body to see what it needs (or should avoid). As Anna Lappé and I stressed in our book *Grub: Ideas for an Urban Organic Kitchen*, "We all have specific body constitutions, cultural foodways, and personal tastes that determine which foods work for us. No single way of eating is perfect for everyone. In fact, because our bodies are so dynamic, no single diet is perfect for any one throughout her or his life. Our relationship with food should be fluid, shifting as we change."

To be clear, though, I am not presenting this as a "healthy cookbook." *Vegan Soul Kitchen* is a *real food* cookbook for *anyone with soul* that likes tasty eats. While there are books that present low-calorie, low-fat, no-fat, and salt-free versions of African American and Southern cooking, many of them still suggest unhealthy ingredients

such as denatured white sugar, acrid table salt, genetically modified fats, refined grains, processed flours, and sometimes canned food items.

Rather than counting calories, sacrificing flavor-enhancing ingredients like salt and "good" fat, and recommending unhealthy industrial ingredients, *Vegan Soul Kitchen* offers animal-product-free recipes mostly inspired by African American and Southern cuisine that use fresh, whole, best-quality, health-supportive ingredients and healthful cooking techniques with an eye on local, seasonal, sustainably grown real food. This cookbook also provides a much-needed intervention in a genre oversaturated with books that include animal products. It's easy to insert meat or dairy products in many of these dishes if that's what you need. So feel free to add, omit, or substitute suggested ingredients to make these recipes work for you. Freestyle and be creative. 'Cause I was.

Here, I have imagined new recipes through the prism of the African diaspora—cutting, pasting, reworking, and remixing African, Caribbean, African American, Native American, and European staples, cooking techniques, and distinctive dishes to come up with something all my own. Like a DJ being moved by the energy of the crowd to guide selections, I let the spirits of my ancestors and progeny move me to conjure up these edible treats. African American food historian Jessica B. Harris contends that this way with food is a "microcosm of our history."[3] I would add that this approach encapsulates our future as well.

Through recipes like **Uncle Don's Double Mustard Greens and Roasted Yam Soup**; **Cajun-Creole-Spiced Tempeh Pieces with Creamy Grits**; **Caramelized Grapefruit, Avocado, and Watercress Salad with Grapefruit Vinaigrette**; and **Sweet Cornmeal-Coconut Butter Drop Biscuits** I am pushing the boundaries of what we understand as African American and Southern cuisine.

More than anything, I hope to return our focus to fresh, whole, local, seasonal, and sustainably grown *real food* and away from what author Michael Pollan calls "edible foodlike substances" (processed, canned, packaged, fast, and industrial).[4]

Think: Alice Waters meets Melvin Van Peebles. To complement the pleasures that you will derive from the prepared recipes, I offer a beautiful prayer-song written by my uncle Don Bryant and a moving poem by Michael Molina; I include my signature "suggested soundtrack"—either an individual song or a whole album—with every recipe (to be enjoyed while cooking and eating); I recommend films, books, and visual artwork; and I incorporate photographs of several dishes taken by the amazingly brilliant Sara Remington as well as an image by Keba Konte and one by Brittany M. Powell. It is my intention to help bring the "culture back in agriculture," as Chef Dan Barber would say.

I also hope that *Vegan Soul Kitchen* helps shift African American cuisine back to our home gardens and kitchens. My grandparents raised their own chickens, kept gardens that produced most of their vegetables, and maintained mini-orchards in their front and backyards. Several of their neighbors did the same. Now the fowl, plots, and fruit trees have disappeared from their South Memphis neighborhood. And many of the denizens of this community are suffering from hypertension, diabetes, and other often preventable, diet-related illnesses. My memory of a "greener" South, as explored in my essay "Reclaiming True Grits," reawakened my desire to write this book to help people remember that part of our legacy.[5] Like most Americans, African Americans saw the globalization of agriculture and industrialization of food as a good

3. Jessica B. Harris, *The Welcome Table: African-American Heritage Cooking* (New York: Fireside, 1995).

4. Michael Pollan, *In Defense of Food: An Eater's Manifesto* (New York: Penguin, 2008).

5. Bryant Terry, "Reclaiming True Grits," theroot .com. Accessed online October 12, 2008, at http:// www.theroot.com/id/45056/page/1.

thing. Cheap. Fast. Convenient. It all seemed to make sense. But today we recognize the fallout from that food system—on our bodies, spirits, cultures, and communities—and it's time now to get back to the land. And celebrate!

These recipes were composed with my desire to bring festive food back to the center of pleasurable community building and cultural celebration with weekends, dinner parties, cookouts, and special occasions in mind. So explore the food, words, images, and music. Shake ya a**, watch ya self, and getcha grub on!

Bryant Terry

RAISE YOUR STOCK
ESSENTIAL GEAR FOR YOUR KITCHEN

So here's the deal. There is some kitchen gear that can make all the difference in the level of ease with which you make a lot of recipes in this book (and in general). So I'm going to offer suggestions. But I would invite you to use your creativity and improvise when you don't have certain equipment. It took me several years to raise my own stock, so consider what is a priority for you to purchase immediately, and freestyle as you go.

Baking Dishes: Keep a few 2-quart glass baking dishes handy.

Baking Sheets: two baking sheets are sufficient for all my needs.

Blender: I use my upright blender almost every day, mostly for making smoothies and sometimes for blending salad dressings and pureeing creamy soups. I also own an immersion blender—a handheld electric wand-shaped device with a blade at the bottom—but I typically only use it when I am pureeing a huge batch of soup. Call me old-fashioned but there is something rewarding about the process of ladling a soup into a traditional blender and pureeing it in batches (when cooking for two to four people).

Bowls: Nowadays, you can easily find inexpensive sets of stainless-steel mixing bowls. And if you want to be fancy, you can purchase a set of porcelain mixing bowls. Both kinds come in handy when making dishes that require lots of prepped ingredients. I also use them to hold food in the refrigerator (while it is cooling, marinating, and the like). They store easily when you buy them in a stackable nest.

Canning Jars: I keep three different sizes handy: half-pint, pint, and quart. In addition to using them for preserves and pickles, I store spices, beans, grains, and leftover food in them. I also use them for serving drinks.

Cheesecloth: Cheesecloth is great for straining broths, squeezing seedless juice from citrus fruits, extracting juice from grated ginger pulp, making nut milks, and extracting strawberry nectar from fresh strawberries.

Coffee/Spice Grinder: I prefer using a mortar and pestle to pulverize most spices, but an electric grinder is best for harder to grind spices like cinnamon sticks, dried chipotle chile, and whole cloves. Unless you want coffee-flavored spices or spice-flavored coffee (it's actually tasty), use a separate grinder for coffee beans and spices.

Colander: I keep a large colander handy for draining vegetables.

Cutting Board: To avoid cross-contamination (if you cook with animal products) and transferal of onion and garlic flavors to fruits, I recommend keeping a few cutting boards in your kitchen. I keep three: a thick wooden cutting board for vegetables, a smaller wooden cutting board for fruits, and a black plastic cutting board for seafood. Remember to "season" your wooden cutting boards with oil (use a USP-grade mineral oil) after washing to prevent them from drying out and buckling.

Food Processor: While I have always used my food processor for making dips, spreads, and pie fillings, I just recently started using it as a timesaving tool for prepping vegeta-bles. I used to romanticize "communing with the ingredients" (actually I still do), but when I'm pressed for time I pull out those handy attachments that came with my food processor and let technology do all the work.

Grater: I use my four-sided box grater to shred vegetables and fruits.

Kitchen Timer: My timer has saved me many a time from overcooking a dish because I'm preoccupied with something else. It also helps when you are watching the time for more than one dish.

Knives: I highly recommend investing in a good chef's knife (you can usually find them on sale around the Christmas holiday). It is best to comparison shop and try out several to see which one feels most comfortable in your hand. If you take good care of it, your chef's knife should last you a long time. I have two: an 8-inch Japanese chef's knife and an 8-inch French chef's knife. I also keep a 10-inch serrated knife for cutting bread and a small serrated knife (my favorite) for cutting tomatoes and citrus fruits. I learned a long time ago that knives don't cut people, dull knives cut people (mostly because they don't slice cleanly through food). So invest in a steel for daily sharpening and a stone for honing the blade when it gets dull.

Ladles: A 6–8-ounce ladle usually serves all of my kitchen needs.

Measuring Cups and Spoons: I keep good-quality metal measuring cups and spoons on hand for dry goods and sturdy glass measures on hand for liquids.

Microplane Grater/Zester: A microplane is great for zesting citrus fruits without cutting into the white pith. They also generate fluffy pieces of chocolate.

Mortar and Pestle: I actually collect mortar and pestles. So far, I have about eighteen from twelve different countries. They are great for grinding spices and making guacamole and pesto.

Parchment Paper: Parchment paper usually decreases the fat needed to cook food in the oven and it prevents food from sticking to baking sheets and roasting pans, thereby extending their usage life.

Peeler: There are many types of peelers on the market, but I find that a solid Y-shaped swivel peeler tends to hold up the longest and get the job done the best. Not only do I use it for peeling the skin off of vegetables and fruits, but I also shave strips of vegetables for salads and stir-fries with it. Similar to your kitchen knives, it's best to go to a kitchen supply store and "test drive" a

number of peelers and see which ones feel most comfortable in your hands.

Pepper Mill: Similar to other spices, freshly ground pepper is a lot more flavorful and aromatic than preground. Buying whole peppercorns and grinding them just before adding to a dish will ensure that you have the strongest flavors. Make sure you add pepper right at the end of cooking since it loses its flavor and aroma if cooked for too long.

Pots and Pans: Investing in quality cookware is one way that I practice sustainability. Rather than purchasing less expensive pieces that will have to be replaced in a few years, I buy best-quality pots and pans that will last a lifetime with proper care (and that come with a lifetime warranty). If you read my blog entries, you already know I stan for All-Clad. There are less expensive brands that get the job done, but All-Clad is the Maybach of cookware. And they sell great sets to serve many of your cooking needs. That being said, if you will be purchasing your pieces separately I suggest the following to get you started:

- 10-inch fry pan
- 4-quart saucepan with lid
- 3-quart sauté pan with lid
- 7-quart stockpot with lid

Salad Spinner: A good-quality salad spinner is indispensable. If you don't dry your salad greens adequately after washing them, the clinging water will prevent the salad dressing from coating the leaves, and the flavor will be diluted.

Sieves: I use a medium-mesh sieve for straining pureed soups. They also come in handy for draining small quantities of vegetables, beans, and grains.

Spatula: I keep two types of spatulas handy: a rubber spatula for scraping ingredients out of bowls and folding together wet and dry ingredients and a wooden spatula for turning ingredients when they are being sautéed.

Spider: Kinda like a sieve with a long wooden handle attached. I use my spider often for deep-frying and removing ingredients from boiling liquids.

Spoons: Whenever I am stirring sauces or sautéing I use wooden spoons.

Tongs: Tongs are essential for grilling. They are also good for turning tofu, tempeh, and seitan when you are sautéing and frying them.

Whisks: A large stainless-steel whisk comes in handy for making vinaigrettes and grits and for preparing ingredients for baking.

THE
GRUB

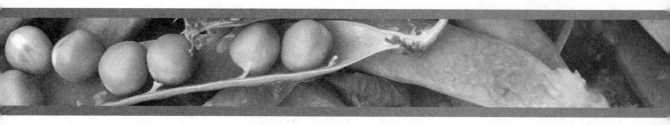

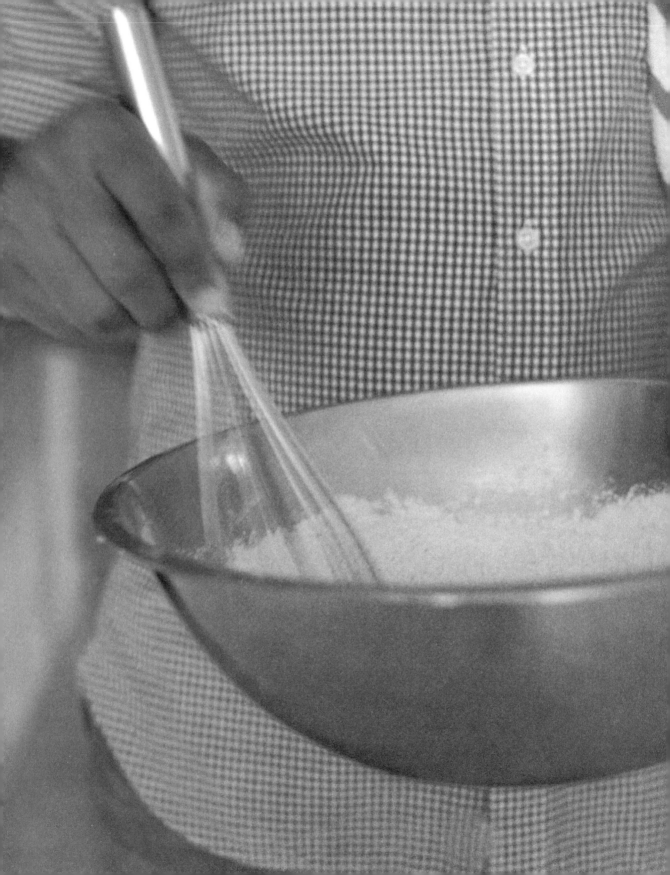

TOP SIX GOOD EATS
YOU GOTTA REWIND ME

- Citrus Collards with Raisins Redux •

• Agave-Sweetened Orange-Orange Pekoe Tea •

• Sweet Sweetback's Salad with
Roasted Beet Vinaigrette •

• Uncle Don's Double Mustard Greens
and Roasted Yam Soup •

• Cajun-Creole-Spiced Tempeh Pieces with Creamy Grits •

• Open-Faced BBQ Tempeh Sandwich with Carrot-Cayenne Coleslaw •

It's what you all been waitin' for ain't it?
What people pay paper for damn it.

—Kanye West, "Barry Bonds"

People often ask, "What is your favorite recipe in this book?" For me, answering that question is kinda like choosing a favorite child, as all of these dishes have a special place in my heart and belly. But there are a few that stand out.

Inspired by chef Jamie Oliver's "Top Ten" in his cookbook *Jamie's Dinners*, here I highlight six dishes included in this book that reflect the spirit of cutting, pasting, reworking, and remixing African, Caribbean, African American, Native American, and European staples, cooking techniques, and distinctive dishes to come up with something all my own. I'm sure you will be rewinding back to these often.

CITRUS COLLARDS WITH RAISINS REDUX

Yield: 4 servings

Soundtrack: "Sankofa" by Hypnotic Brass Ensemble and Tony Allen from *Allen Chop Up* and "Sankofa" by Cassandra Wilson from *Blue Light 'Til Dawn*

This recipe was the seed of *Vegan Soul Kitchen* . . . a brand new classic, if you will, dedicated to my home city in the mid-South—Memphis, Tennessee.

Coarse sea salt

2 large bunches collard greens, ribs removed, cut into a chiffonade, rinsed and drained (pages 4 and page 8).

1 tablespoon extra-virgin olive oil

2 cloves garlic, minced

2/3 cup raisins

1/3 cup freshly squeezed orange juice

- In a large pot over high heat, bring 3 quarts of water to a boil and add 1 tablespoon salt. Add the collards and cook, uncovered, for 8 to 10 minutes, until softened. Meanwhile, prepare a large bowl of ice water to cool the collards.

- Remove the collards from the heat, drain, and plunge them into the bowl of cold water to stop cooking and set the color of the greens. Drain by gently pressing the greens against a colander.

- In a medium-size sauté pan, combine the olive oil and the garlic and raise the heat to medium. Sauté for 1 minute. Add the collards, raisins, and 1/2 teaspoon salt. Sauté for 3 minutes, stirring frequently.

- Add orange juice and cook for an additional 15 seconds. Do not overcook (collards should be bright green). Season with additional salt to taste if needed and serve immediately. (This also makes a tasty filling for quesadillas.)

CHIFFONADE

The chiffonade cut is used to produce very fine threads of leafy fresh herbs as well as greens and other leafy vegetables. First, remove any tough stems that would prevent the leaf from being rolled tightly (reserve them for stocks or salads). Next, stack several leaves, roll them widthwise into a tight cylinder, and slice crosswise with a sharp knife, cutting the leaves into thin strips.

AGAVE-SWEETENED ORANGE-ORANGE PEKOE TEA

Yield: 12 to 14 servings
Soundtrack: "Mississippi Goddamn" by Nina Simone from *Protest Anthology*

Ma'Dear, my maternal grandmother, would sun-brew gallon jars full of Sweet Goodness on sweltering hot summer days. Recollections of those containers full of cinnamon-colored tea sitting on her back porch bring back sweet memories of simpler days. This version will satisfy the snootiest of Sweet Tea connoisseurs (read: my mom) and won't give drinkers an insulin spike since it is sweetened with agave nectar.

12 cups cold water
2 2-inch cinnamon sticks
12 tea bags orange-flavored black tea
2 cups freshly squeezed orange juice
1/2 cup freshly squeezed lemon juice
1 1/2 cups agave nectar
Ice cubes
Thin orange wedges, for garnish

- In a stockpot, combine the water and cinnamon sticks and bring to a boil. Remove from heat and immediately add the tea bags, orange juice, lemon juice, and agave nectar. Cover and let stand for 30 minutes.
- Remove the lid, allow the tea to cool, and remove the tea bags with a slotted spoon.
- To serve, ladle into pint-size canning jars filled with ice and garnish with orange wedges.

ORANGE JUICE

If you like the flavor of commercial orange juice, drink it 'til your palate is content, but if you're looking for nutrients you might want to look elsewhere. My friend and colleague Alissa Hamilton, author of *Squeezed: What You Don't Know about Orange Juice* (Yale University Press, 2009), explains: "If vitamin C is really what you are after, you'd be better off eating a whole orange than drinking a glass of juice. In fact, you would be best off with a handful of sliced red peppers, which are almost four times as high in vitamin C as oranges. Brussels sprouts, broccoli, guava, kiwi, papaya and strawberries also all top citrus when it comes to vitamin C."

SWEET SWEETBACK'S SALAD WITH ROASTED BEET VINAIGRETTE

Yield: 4 to 6 servings

Soundtrack (all songs that contain samples of Melvin Van Peebles' music): "30 Cops or More" by Boogie Down Productions from *Edutainment;* "The Finest" by MF DOOM from *Operation Doomsday;* "Come on Feet" by Quasimoto from *The Unseen;* "Hydrant Game" by Quasimoto from *The Further Adventures of Lord Quas*

Film: *How to Eat Your Watermelon in White Company (and Enjoy It)* (2005), directed by Joe Angio. This documentary chronicles Melvin Van Peebles' astonishing career.

In March 2008 I went to Los Angeles to film an episode for *MVP's Greenhouse*, a television series that follows Mario Van Peebles, his wife, their five children, and his father (Melvin Van Peebles) as they renovate their LA home in an environmentally friendly manner and embrace a more sustainable lifestyle. I was excited to help Mario prepare a meal, but I was overjoyed to be in the presence of Melvin.

I created this salad not so much in honor of Melvin's cult classic *Sweet Sweetback's Baadasssss Song* or the moving biopic—*Baadasssss*—written and directed by Mario, but more so for Melvin's influence on me as a creative person. In addition to being a screenwriter, director, actor, and film editor, Melvin's creative pursuits include being a painter, sculptor, children's book author, dancer, novelist, journalist, translator, composer, recording artist, playwright, playboy, Broadway producer, and stockbroker (the first African American to hold a seat on the American Stock Exchange). And at seventy-seven years old he's still going strong. Black genius indeed.

Like Sweetback, the protagonist of *Sweet Sweetback's Baadasssss Song,* this salad is bold (beets), bitter (arugula), earthy (walnuts), and sweet (agave nectar).

4 medium beets, scrubbed, tops trimmed, root tails left intact

Coarse sea salt

4 tablespoons plus 4 teaspoons extra-virgin olive oil

3 tablespoons red wine vinegar

1/2 teaspoon Dijon mustard

1/2 teaspoon agave nectar

Freshly ground white pepper

3 large bunches arugula, trimmed and roughly chopped (6 to 7 cups)

1 1/2 cups **Candied Walnuts** (page 40)

- Combine the beets, 3 quarts cold water, and 1 teaspoon salt in a medium pot over high heat. Boil uncovered for 20 to 30 minutes, or until the beets are easily pierced with a knife. Drain. Peel the beets by holding them under cold running water and rubbing their skins off with your fingers or a clean towel.

- Preheat oven to 400°F.

- Trim the tails off the bottom of the beets. Reserve two of them for the vinaigrette and compost the others. Cut the beets into 1/4-inch dice. In a medium bowl, toss the diced beets with 4 teaspoons of the olive oil. Transfer them to a parchment-lined baking sheet and roast for 15 minutes, stirring every 5 minutes to ensure even cooking. Remove the beets from the oven, transfer them back into the bowl just used, and toss with 2 tablespoons of red wine vinegar. Return to the baking sheet and cook for an additional 5 minutes. Set them aside to cool.

- In a blender, combine the reserved roasted beet tails with the remaining red wine vinegar, mustard, agave nectar, 1/4 teaspoon salt, and white pepper to taste. Blend while slowly pouring in 4 tablespoons of olive oil. If needed, add more salt to taste.

- Place the arugula pieces in a large serving bowl, add the roasted beets on top, and add the candied walnuts on top of that. Immediately before serving, toss well with just enough of the vinaigrette to coat.

UNCLE DON'S DOUBLE MUSTARD GREENS AND ROASTED YAM SOUP

Yield: 4 to 6 servings
Soundtrack: "I Can't Stand the Rain" by Ann Peebles from *Brand New Classics*

Every time I sit down for a meal I express gratitude for all the forces that helped bring the food to my plate: the natural elements, farmers, farmhands, transporters, chefs, kitchen assistants, and servers in many cases. Because I want to encourage others to do so as well, I asked my Uncle Don Bryant (my first name is my mother's maiden name) if he would compose an original prayer-song to contribute. As you saw at the beginning of the book, he said yes!

Uncle Don was a well-known songwriter-singer in the 1970s. He was the staff songwriter at Hi Records, and he penned a slew of hits for that label's artists (including Al Green, Willie Mitchell, and Ann Peebles). His most celebrated songs were written for his wife, Ann Peebles. You know that song "I Can't Stand the Rain," which was covered by over thirty artists (including Cassandra Wilson, Michael Bolton, and Tina Turner) and sampled by Missy Elliott for her first big hit "The Rain (Supa Dupa Fly)"? Well, Uncle Don wrote it.

To show my gratitude, I created this soup in his honor.

CLEANING GREENS

I find that cutting greens into the desired size for the dish that I am preparing makes them easier to clean. After thoroughly washing your sink (or a large bowl) of any residue, plug the drain, add the greens, and run cold water until the greens are submerged, agitating them as the sink fills up. Turn off the water and let the greens sit for a minute or so. Next, lift them from the sink with your hands into a large bowl or similar receptacle. Drain the sink of its water, and repeat until the bottom of the sink is free of any residue. Transfer the greens to a colander and drain. Obviously, if you clean delicate leaves like lettuce you want to dry them in a salad spinner.

1 large garnet yam (about 1 pound), peeled and cut into 1/2-inch chunks

2 tablespoons extra-virgin olive oil

Coarse sea salt

4 cups **Simple Stock** (see page 76)

1 large bunch mustard greens (about 1 pound), tough stems removed, chopped into bite-size pieces, washed, and drained

1 teaspoon mustard seeds

3 cloves garlic, minced

2 teaspoons apple cider vinegar

White pepper

- Preheat the oven to 425°F.

- In a large bowl, toss the yams with 1 tablespoon of the olive oil and 1/4 teaspoon of the salt. Transfer the yams to a parchment-lined baking dish and roast for 1 hour, stirring every 15 minutes, until they are starting to crisp on the edges.

- While the yams are roasting, bring the stock to a boil in a medium-size saucepan over high heat. Add the mustard greens and cook, uncovered, for 4 to 6 minutes, until softened. Remove the greens from the heat, drain the stock into a bowl, and set aside. Set the greens aside in a colander.

- Over medium heat in the saucepan just used, warm 1 tablespoon of the olive oil. Add the mustard seeds and cook, stirring occasionally, until they start to pop, 2 to 3 minutes. Next add the garlic and sauté until fragrant, about 1 1/2 minutes. Then add the greens and 1/4 teaspoon salt. Sauté the greens, stirring occasionally, until most of the liquid has evaporated, about 3 minutes. Add the stock back to the saucepan and set aside.

- When the yams are done, transfer them to the saucepan. Bring to a boil, then lower the heat to medium and simmer for about 25 minutes, until the yams are fork tender. Add the apple cider vinegar and white pepper and additional salt to taste.

CAJUN-CREOLE-SPICED TEMPEH PIECES WITH CREAMY GRITS

Yield: 4 to 6 servings
Soundtrack: "A Love Supreme" by Alice Coltrane from *World Galaxy* and "A Love Supreme" by John Coltrane from *A Love Supreme*

On Valentine's Day 2008 my fiancée and I had dinner at Farmer Brown Restaurant in San Francisco, where my friend Jay Foster, the chef-owner, serves up some slammin' "farm-fresh soul food," including Cajun Shrimp with Creamy Grits. Here I reinterpret that dish, incorporating creamed cashews into the grits to give them the velvety texture that usually comes from heavy cream and sautéing then spicing tempeh that was simmered in Simple Stock to replace the shrimp.

Cajun-Creole-Spiced Tempeh

1/2 pound (1 8-ounce package) tempeh
4 cups **Simple Stock** (page 76)
1 teaspoon fine sea salt
1 teaspoon onion powder
2 teaspoons garlic powder
1 teaspoon paprika
1 teaspoon chili powder
1 teaspoon red pepper flakes
1/4 teaspoon cayenne
1 teaspoon dried thyme
1 teaspoon dried oregano
1 teaspoon freshly ground white pepper
1/2 cup extra-virgin olive oil, plus more for frying if needed

Grits

1 pint cherry tomatoes, stemmed and quartered
2 tablespoons freshly squeezed lemon juice
1/2 teaspoon fine sea salt
1 tablespoon extra-virgin olive oil
1 medium leek (white and tender green parts), chopped finely (about 3/4 cup)
2 cloves garlic, minced
2 1/2 cups water
1 cup **Simple Stock** (page 76)
3/4 cup stone-ground grits
1 cup **Almond Milk** (page 28) or unflavored rice milk
1/2 cup **Creamed Cashews** (page 168)
1 scallion, sliced thinly, for garnish

For the tempeh

- Cut the tempeh into 1/2-inch fingers. Cut those fingers in half lengthwise, and cut those pieces in half widthwise.

- In a medium-size saucepan, combine the Simple Stock and 1/2 teaspoon salt. Stir until the salt is dissolved, then add the tempeh pieces. Bring to a boil, lower the heat to medium-high, cover, and simmer for 25 minutes, until the tempeh is moist and saturated with vegetable broth. Remove from the heat, drain the tempeh in a colander (reserving the stock for later use), and let the pieces dry for about 30 minutes.

- In a medium-size paper bag, combine the onion powder, garlic powder, paprika, chili powder, red pepper flakes, cayenne, thyme, oregano, white pepper, and 1/4 teaspoon salt. Fold the top of the bag over a few times and shake well until combined. Open the top and set aside.

- In a large skillet over medium-high heat, warm the olive oil. Add the tempeh pieces and cook for 2 to 3 minutes, until golden brown on the bottom. With a fork, turn the fingers over and cook for 2 to 3 more minutes, until golden brown. With a slotted spoon, *immediately* transfer all the tempeh pieces to the paper bag with the dried spices and herbs. Fold the bag over a few times to close and shake vigorously until all pieces are coated well with the seasoning, about 1 minute.

For the grits

- While the tempeh is simmering, combine the tomatoes, lemon juice, and 1/4 teaspoon salt in a bowl and toss well. Cover and refrigerate.

- In a large skillet over medium heat, combine the olive oil with the leek and sauté, stirring a few times, until browned, about 2 to 3 minutes. Add the garlic and cook until fragrant. Transfer mixture to a medium-size bowl and set aside.

- To prepare the grits, in a medium-size saucepan, combine 2 cups of water, the Simple Stock, and 1/2 teaspoon salt and bring to a boil. Whisk the grits into the liquid until no lumps remain, return to a boil, then quickly reduce the heat to low and simmer, stirring frequently to prevent the grits from sticking to the bottom of the pan, until the grits have absorbed most of the liquid and are thickening, 10 to 12 minutes. Stir in the Almond Milk and simmer for another 10 minutes, stirring frequently, until most of the liquid has been absorbed. Stir in the Creamed Cashews and the remaining 1/2 cup water and simmer, stirring frequently, until the grits are soft but not runny, about 35 to 40 minutes.

- Remove the tomatoes from the refrigerator, drain them of their juices, and transfer to the bowl with the leek mixture. Add the tempeh pieces and mix well.

- For each serving, spoon about 1/2 cup of the tempeh mixture over 3/4 cup of grits. Garnish with scallions.

OPEN-FACED BBQ TEMPEH SANDWICH WITH CARROT-CAYENNE COLESLAW

Yield: 5 servings
Soundtrack: "Packt Like Sardines in a Crushed Tin Box" by Radiohead from *Amnesiac*

I created this sandwich in July 2007 for "Pit Stop," an event celebrating the twentieth anniversary of the Berkeley Farmers' Markets (get it, barbecue pit/peach pit). This tempeh recipe is an adaptation from a recipe included in one my favorite cookbooks—*The Modern Vegetarian Kitchen* by Peter Berley. Instead of a regular bun, I served the coleslaw and tempeh fingers atop focaccia that was donated by a local bakery. The sandwiches were a big hit with vegans, vegetarians, and meat eaters alike.

If you aren't grilling it you can pack the tempeh in a baking dish, cover with the barbecue sauce, and bake at 350°F for 1 hour.

TEMPEH

Originally from Indonesia, tempeh is a dense, fermented soybean cake that has a subtle, nutty flavor. When I hear people complain about the "blandness" of tempeh, I assume that they have not had it cooked properly. There are three primary ways that I add flavor to tempeh. I fry it in fat and then sprinkle it with sea salt (e.g., **Pan-Fried Coconut-Tempeh Cubes with Creamy Celeriac Sauce**, page 50); I simmer it on a stove in a light broth or stock (e.g., **Good Green Tempeh Packet,** page 151); or I oven-bake it covered in a marinade or sauce (e.g., **Open-Faced BBQ Tempeh Sandwiches with Carrot-Cayenne Coleslaw**, above). Using these basic cooking techniques, you can be sure to have tasty tempeh without fear of the "B" word. While there are several commercial brands on the market, my favorite is Lightlife.

3 tablespoons apple cider vinegar

3 tablespoons freshly squeezed
lime juice

3/4 cup tamari

1/4 cup canned tomato sauce

1 large chipotle chile in adobo sauce

3 tablespoons extra-virgin olive oil

1/4 cup agave nectar

1 tablespoon ground cumin

1/8 teaspoon cayenne

2 tablespoons water

1 pound tempeh (2 8-ounce packages),
cut into 1/2 inch fingers

5 4 x 4-inch pieces of focaccia

4 1/2 cups **Carrot-Cayenne Coleslaw**
(page 63)

- In a blender, combine the apple cider vinegar, lime juice, tamari, tomato sauce, chile, olive oil, agave nectar, cumin, cayenne, and water to create a marinade. Puree until well combined. Set aside.

- Preheat grill.

- In a large baking dish, place the tempeh fingers in one snug layer. Pour the marinade on them and tightly cover the dish with foil. Transfer to the grill, close, and bake for 50 minutes, turning the tempeh once halfway through.

- Remove the baking dish from the grill. With a slotted spoon, transfer the tempeh fingers back to the grill and cook until sizzling and slightly charred, about 1 minute per side.

- While the tempeh is grilling, put the focaccia on the grill and cook until warm and slightly charred, about 2 minutes per side.

- Construct the sandwiches by adding 3 to 4 tempeh fingers to each square of focaccia and topping with coleslaw.

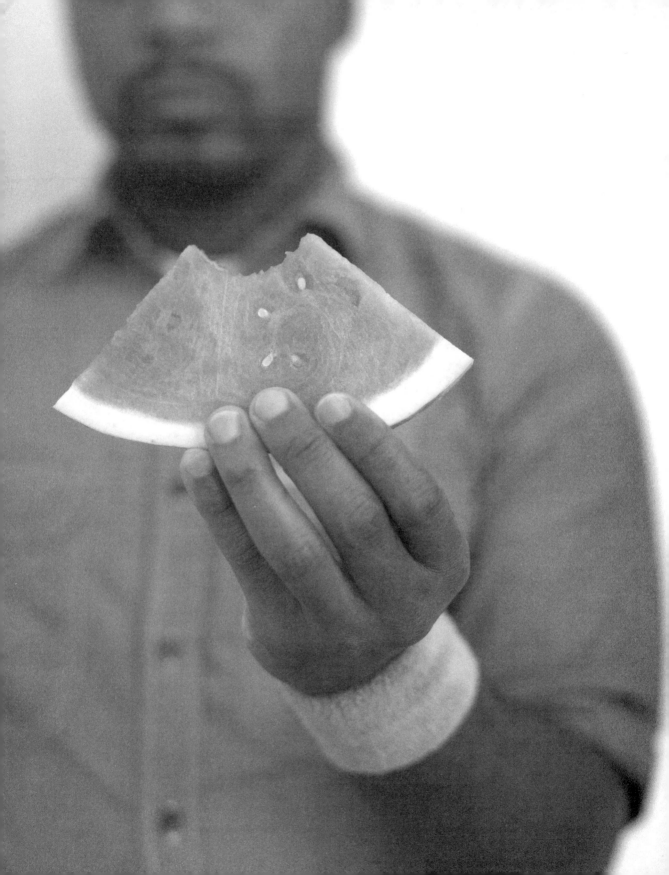

IT'S ALL GOOD
ZERO-WASTE WATERMELON

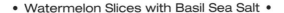

• Watermelon Slices with Basil Sea Salt •

• Fresh Watermelon–Vodka Martini •

• Double Watermelon–Strawberry Slushee •

• Red-Rocket Salad with Watermelon-Basil Vinaigrette •

• Citrus and Spice Pickled Watermelon Rind •

• Balsamic Syrup–Sweetened Watermelon Sorbet •

It's one thing for me to talk and write about maintaining sustainable habits, and it is another to actually live them out. So before we get to the main section of this book, I want to illustrate how I am constantly searching for creative ways to practice eco-sustainability in my own life. I always try to use as many parts of fruits and vegetables as possible before composting. For example, I reserve the tough parts and trimmings of vegetables to make **Simple Stock** (page 76); I scoop the seeds out of winter squashes, toss them in a little extra-virgin olive oil and spices, and cook them in the oven to make **Roasted Winter Squash Seeds** (page 43); and I slice the spines of collard greens and sauté them with olive oil, lemon juice, and salt to make **Collard Confetti** (page 118).

I especially like experimenting with fruits. My fascination with working with the different components of them started when I had over a dozen whole blood orange peels after making my **Blood Orange Sorbet** (from *Grub*). I combined half of the peels with fresh mint and water to make **Citrus Zest and Fresh Mint Tea** (page 27), and I used the rest to make **Candied Orange Peel** (page 189). Here I use one of my favorite fruits, watermelon, and illustrate the numerous ways in which one can make the most of all its parts.

WATERMELON SLICES WITH BASIL SEA SALT

Yield: 4 servings

Soundtrack: "Watermelon Man" by Herbie Hancock from *Head Hunters*

Film: *Watermelon Man* (1970), directed by Melvin Van Peebles. This narrative film tells the story of a white insurance salesman who wakes up one morning to find that he has become black.

Although many of my family members would add a dash of salt to fresh watermelon when I was young, I would always pass. Why would you ruin perfectly sweet watermelon with salt? Now I know that a tad of salt actually adds a pleasant contrast and helps bring out some of the watermelon's sweetness. Basil, which goes perfectly with watermelon, provides a nice accent.

8 slices of ripe yellow or red watermelon (or a mix)

Herbed Sea Salt (basil) (page 162)

- Sprinkle the watermelon with the basil salt and serve each guest two slices.

WATERMELON JUICE AND WATERMELON WATER

To make watermelon juice, add watermelon chunks to an upright blender, puree until liquefied, and then strain through a fine-mesh sieve to remove all solids. (Compost the pulp.) Every 3 pounds of watermelon (before the rind is removed) usually yields between 3½ to 4 cups of juice, after straining.

Besides drinking the tasty juice of watermelons straight and using it to make drinks, watermelon vinaigrette, watermelon popsicles, and sorbet, I add it to water to give it a fruity essence. Use 1 part watermelon juice for every 6 parts of water.

FRESH WATERMELON–VODKA MARTINI

Yield: 2 servings
Soundtrack: "Who Me?" by KMD from *The Best of KMD*
Art: "How to Market Kitty Litter to Black People" by Hank Willis Thomas

Because of the racial stereotypes associated with black folks eating watermelon, I intentionally avoided it throughout most of my adolescent years. Now I eat it all the time. Here's to eating (and drinking) watermelon and enjoying it (clink, clink).

ORGANIC SPIRITS AND WINE

While I certainly would not suggest having alcoholic beverages often (they are high in sugar content), I'm all about moderately enjoying wine and mixing up creative cocktails at dinner parties and cookouts. Since I have expanded my environmental stewardship efforts to include spirits and wines that I choose to buy, I seek out organic or biodynamic alcoholic beverages made with grains and fruits grown in a way that does not negatively impact the environment.

1 tablespoon freshly squeezed lime juice

1 tablespoon freshly squeezed orange juice

1 tablespoon agave nectar

6 tablespoons vodka

1/2 cup fresh red watermelon juice (page 16)

2 red watermelon wedges (with rind), 2 inches long and 1/2 inch thick

Herbed Sea Salt (basil) (page 162)

- Fill a cocktail shaker with ice. Top it with cold water, and place in a freezer. Next, rinse two martini glasses with cold water and immediately place them in a freezer.
- Remove cocktail shaker from the freezer, empty, and refill with fresh ice.
- Add the lime juice, orange juice, agave nectar, vodka, and watermelon juice in the chilled cocktail shaker. Vigorously shake ingredients until well chilled, about 30 seconds. Strain into the martini glass. Garnish with a wedge of watermelon by placing it directly in the martini glass (with the rind sticking out), add a pinch of Basil Sea Salt, and serve.

DOUBLE WATERMELON–STRAWBERRY SLUSHEE

Yield: 4 to 6 servings

Soundtrack: "Back and Forth" by Aaliyah from *Age Ain't Nothing but a Number* and "Black Mags" by The Cool Kids from *The Bake Sale*

Takin' y'all back and forward at the same time. Feel me?

----

8 cups fresh red watermelon juice
   (page 16)

2 cups frozen strawberries

2 tablespoons freshly squeezed
   lime juice

¼ cup agave nectar

4–6 fresh mint sprigs, for garnish

- Fill two large ice cube trays with watermelon juice and freeze until solid, 3 to 4 hours.
- In an upright blender, combine 1 full tray of watermelon cubes, 2 cups of watermelon juice, and 1 cup of frozen strawberries (the blender should be full). Blend on high speed until well-combined and slushy, about 1 minute. Add 1 tablespoon lime juice and 2 tablespoons agave nectar and blend on high speed for another 30 seconds. Pour into a large pitcher and store in the freezer.
- Repeat.
- Serve immediately in slender clear glasses garnished with mint sprigs.

FREEZING FRUIT FOR SMOOTHIES

I drink lots of smoothies during the summertime, when I transition to lighter fare. First, I freeze fresh seasonal fruit. Next I blend it with filtered water, coconut water, fruit juice, or almond milk until smooth. Most of the time the natural sugars in the fruits are enough, but if I want my smoothie to be sweeter I add one to two pitted dates. Add more to your desired taste.

RED-ROCKET SALAD WITH WATERMELON-BASIL VINAIGRETTE

Yield: 4 servings

Soundtrack: "Rocket Love" by Stevie Wonder from *Hotter than July* and "Rocket Love, Pt. 1" by Yesterdays New Quintet from *Stevie*

Sometimes when I mix vegetables and fruits in the same dish I find that it is harder to digest. Maybe the fact that arugula, also known as rocket, promotes digestion allows me to mix it with fruits and be just fine. This light and refreshing summer salad goes well with a spicy entrée.

1/2 medium seedless watermelon, rind removed, flesh cut into 1/2-inch cubes suitable for presentation (you only need 4 cups)

1/4 cup basil leaves, rough chopped

1 teaspoon freshly squeezed lemon juice

1 cup fresh watermelon juice (page 16)

1 tablespoon apple cider vinegar

1/4 teaspoon Dijon mustard

2 tablespoons minced basil

1/2 teaspoon coarse sea salt

6 tablespoons extra-virgin olive oil

Freshly ground white pepper

2 cups trimmed arugula (rocket)

1/2 cup peanuts, toasted (page 41)

- In a medium bowl, combine the watermelon cubes, basil, and lemon juice, and toss well. Cover and refrigerate.

- In a small saucepan over high heat, bring the watermelon juice to a boil. Lower the heat to medium, simmer, and reduce the juice to 2 tablespoons, 8 to 10 minutes. Immediately transfer to an upright blender and set aside to cool.

- Make the vinaigrette by adding the apple cider vinegar, mustard, basil, and salt to the blender and blending while slowly pouring in the olive oil. Season with white pepper to taste.

- Place the arugula in a medium bowl, add enough vinaigrette to *lightly* coat (reserve the rest for later use), and toss well.

- Divide the dressed arugula evenly among 4 plates, top each salad with 1 cup watermelon cubes, garnish with peanuts, and serve immediately.

CITRUS AND SPICE PICKLED WATERMELON RIND

Yield: 6 pints

Soundtrack: "Water Melon" by Toots & The Maytals from *Toots & The Maytals—Sweet and Dandy—The Best of Toots & The Maytals*

The first thing people say when they try one of these is "Damn that was good, what is it?" It's an-old school Southern classic that I am happy to resuscitate. The recipe takes some commitment, but I guarantee you will be happy you made the effort. I normally eat these as a snack by themselves, but I also have them alongside more savory dishes to provide a sweet contrast (in a similar way that you would enjoy a chutney). And I make a bangin' **Pickled Watermelon Rind Salsa** (page 86).

Rind from a medium-size (10–12 pounds) watermelon (the thicker the better)

3 quarts and 3 cups water

3¼ cups organic raw cane sugar

¾ cup coarse sea salt

4 2-inch cinnamon sticks

2 tablespoons whole cloves

2 large oranges

4 lemons

1 cup apple cider vinegar

1 cup distilled white vinegar

- Prepare the watermelon rinds by removing the green skin with a y-shaped peeler or a utility knife and cutting away most of the red flesh with a knife, but leaving a thin coat (keep them as thick as possible). Next, cut as much of the rind as possible into 1-inch cubes (obviously many of the pieces will be odd shapes) until you generate 10 cups of rind. Set aside.

- In a large stockpot over medium-low heat, make a brine by combining 3 quarts of water with ¼ cup of the sugar, the salt, 2 cinnamon sticks, and 1 tablespoon of cloves. Stir well until the sugar and salt are completely dissolved. Remove from the heat and cool. Transfer the watermelon rind to the brine. Place a small plate on top of the rinds to ensure that they are completely covered in water. Soak overnight.

- Drain the rinds in a colander, and rinse them several times with cold water.

- Combine the rinds with enough cold water to cover them in the stockpot. Bring to a boil, lower heat to medium, then simmer until the pieces are tender but still crisp, about 10 minutes. Drain in a colander and set aside.
- Thinly slice the oranges and the lemons. Combine the vinegars, orange slices, lemon slices, and the remaining sugar, cinnamon sticks, and cloves with the 3 remaining cups of water in the stockpot. Bring to a boil over high heat. Add the rinds, bring back to a boil, reduce the heat to low, cover, and simmer for 10 minutes.
- Drain the rinds in a colander, catching the liquid with a bowl, and set them aside. Add the liquid back to the stockpot, bring to a boil over high heat, and reduce until 4½ cups of liquid remain, 12 to 15 minutes. Transfer the syrup to a metal bowl.
- Preheat the oven to 200°F.
- Bring a large stockpot of water to a boil. Gently place pint-size canning jars, lids, rings, ladles, tongs, and spoons used for canning into the boiling water and simmer for 15 minutes to sterilize. Carefully transfer everything from the stockpot to a baking sheet in the oven until you're ready to start canning.
- Remove baking sheet holding the supplies from the oven. Leaving ½ inch of space at the top, fill the sterilized jars with pieces of watermelon rind, spices, and fruit and then ladle the syrup into each jar. Close the jars with the lids and rings.
- Process in a hot bath for 10 minutes (page 164).

BALSAMIC SYRUP–SWEETENED WATERMELON SORBET

Yield: 3 cups

Soundtrack: "Summertime (UFO Remix)" by Sara Vaughn from *Verve Remixed* and "Summertime" by Miles Davis from *Porgy and Bess*

If you can purchase an ice cream maker, I highly recommend it (most of them are relatively inexpensive these days). Not only do you have control over all of the ingredients that go into your homemade frozen desserts (no gums, preservatives, and the like), but you can also impress your guests with your creative combinations.

If you don't have an ice cream maker, you can easily make this dessert by freezing the mixture overnight in a shallow pan, breaking the mixture up into smaller pieces with a butter knife, and pureeing them in batches in a food processor until slushy.

2 cups balsamic vinegar

2½ cups watermelon juice (page 16)

2 tablespoons agave nectar

2 tablespoons freshly squeezed lemon juice

1 tablespoon vodka (prevents sorbet from freezing all the way)

- In a medium-size saucepan over high heat, bring the balsamic vinegar to a boil. Quickly reduce the heat to medium-low and simmer until the liquid reduces to 3/4 cup, about 30 minutes. Set aside.

- In a container that can be sealed and refrigerated, combine the watermelon juice, agave nectar, lemon juice, and 2 tablespoons of the balsamic syrup (reserve the remaining balsamic syrup and serve over baked potatoes). Stir well to combine and refrigerate until cold.

- Pour into an ice cream maker and freeze until starting to turn slushy, 25 to 30 minutes. Add the vodka and run the machine for an additional 5 minutes. Transfer to an airtight container and place in freezer until firm, about 2 hours.

[THE NAME OF YOUR FAMILY-FAVORITE RECIPE]

Yield: [amount]

I invite you to remix one of your family-favorite recipes. Use it as a guide, modifying it to suit your and (your guests') personal tastes, desires, ethics, politics and dietary restrictions. Freestyle and be creative.

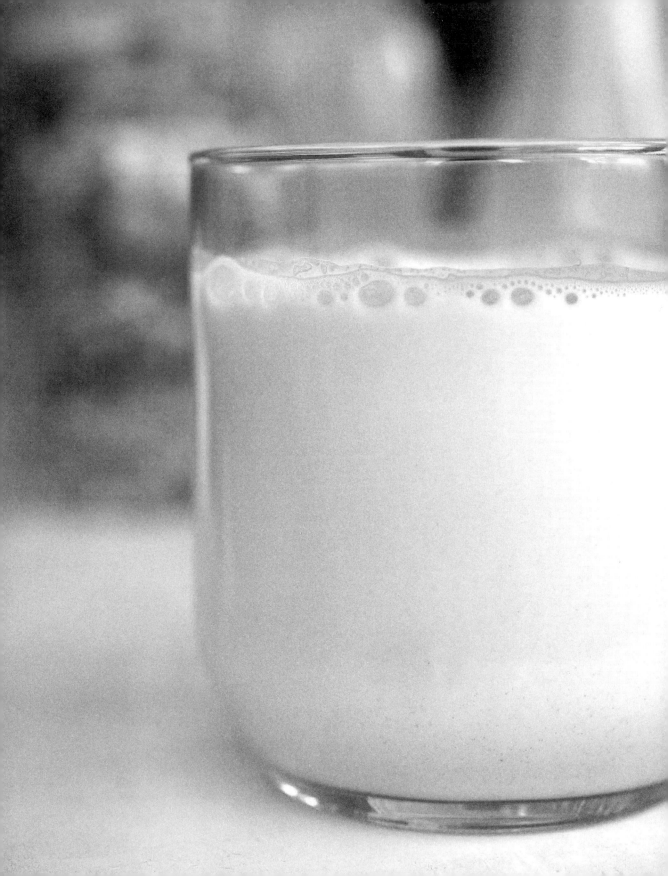

HYDRO GAME
DRINKS

- Simple Syrup •
- Citrus Zest and Fresh Mint Tea •
- Almond Milk •
- Lavender Lemonade •
- Sparkling Rosemary Lemon-Limeade •
- Pure Strawberry Pop •
- Sweet, Sour, and Spicy Blackberry Limeade •
- People's Punch •
- Sin-ger [sin jer] Thirst-Quencher •
- Cinnamon-Applejack Toddy
- California Slurricane •
- Frozen Memphis Mint Julep •

SIMPLE SYRUP

Yield: 2 cups
Soundtrack: "Sugar Water" by Cibo Matto from *Viva! La Woman* and "Sugar Water (Remix)" from *Super Relax*

This simple syrup can be used in place of agave nectar in most cases. It usually can be substituted 1 for 1.

2 cups organic raw cane sugar
1 cup filtered water

* Combine the sugar and the water in a small saucepan over low heat. Stir well until hot to the touch and the sugar is completely dissolved, about 3 minutes. Cool and refrigerate until ready to use.

SWEETENERS

My sweetener of choice, **agave nectar,** is becoming a popular food and beverage sweetener in general, but it is especially good for non–insulin dependent diabetics, as it is a low glycemic index sugar substitute. It's pleasantly sweet, can be used in a range of dishes, and lacks that chemical-ly taste of a lot of chemical sweeteners like Acesulfame-K (Sunette, Sweet & Safe, Sweet One), Aspartame (Equal, Canderel, and NutraSweet), and Sucralose (Splenda). In the past, agave was only available in health food stores, but now many conventional supermarkets carry it as well. My favorite brand is Wholesome Sweeteners, which can be purchased online if you can't find it in a store. When I do use sugar, I opt for organic **raw cane sugar**, which is the least processed of all sugars. I occasionally use **maple crystals**—which are made by evaporating the water from maple syrup—and pure **maple syrup** as well. If a recipe does call for maple syrup, go for certified organic Grade B, which has more nutrients than Grade A.

CITRUS ZEST AND FRESH MINT TEA

Yield: 6 to 8 servings
Soundtrack: "So Fresh, So Clean" by Outkast from *Stankonia*

Fresh herbs infused in water are light, hydrating, and refreshing.

8 cups water

2 large bunches fresh mint, stems removed

Zest strips of 2 organic oranges

Zest strips of 2 organic lemons

1/2 cup agave nectar or **Simple Syrup** (page 26)

Orange slices, for garnish

- In a stockpot, bring the water to a boil. Remove from heat, and immediately stir in the mint, orange zest, lemon zest, and agave nectar. Cover and let stand for 30 minutes.
- Ladle into pint-size canning jars filled with ice and garnish with orange slices.

FLAVORED WATER

A great way to spruce up water is to add slices of naturally cooling and hydrating fruits or vegetables like oranges, lemons, limes, and cucumbers. I only use organic citrus fruits and cucumbers to add to water since their conventional counterparts are treated with toxic chemicals.

ALMOND MILK

Yield: 2 servings
Soundtrack: "Medley: Pastures of
Plenty/This Land Is Your Land/Land"
by Lila Downs from *Border (La Linea)*

I prefer homemade almond milk to
store-bought nut and grains milks for enjoying with cereals, granola, or drinking
straight. I simply find the taste to be much
cleaner. This recipe will last for five days refrigerated. You can use this almond milk in
the recipes in this book where cow's milk
would normally be used, but store-bought
original (unflavored) rice milk can work
with them, too. I generally stay away from
store-bought soy and almond milks, as I find
them to be too sweet and processed-tasting.

1 teaspoon ground cinnamon

$3^{1}/_{2}$ cups filtered water

$1^{1}/_{2}$ cups raw almonds, refrigerated,
soaked in water overnight, and
drained

3 pitted dates

1 teaspoon almond or vanilla extract

- In a small bowl, combine the cinnamon
with 1 tablespoon of the water and mix until well combined. In an upright blender,
combine the almonds, cinnamon-water
slurry, the remaining water, the dates, and
the almond extract. Blend until smooth.
- Strain ingredients through a piece of
cheesecloth into a container that can be
refrigerated, squeezing to extract all of the
liquid.

LAVENDER LEMONADE

Yield: 6 to 8 servings

Soundtrack: "Lavender Woman" by Nat Adderley from *Live at Memory Lane*

In the past I have used lavender to add color, a sweet aroma, and bitter accents to salads, but I have recently started using it in lemonade. The subtle fragrance enlivens this already refreshing beverage.

6 cups water

1/4 cup lavender buds, plus 2 sprigs, for garnish

1/2 cup agave nectar or **Simple Syrup** (page 26)

3/4 cup freshly squeezed lemon juice (from about 6 to 8 lemons)

1 large organic lemon, ends cut off and sliced thinly lengthwise, for garnish

- In a small saucepan, combine 2 cups of the water and the lavender. Bring to a boil, covered, for 10 minutes. Remove from heat and let steep for 10 minutes, then uncover, and set aside to cool.
- Strain the lavender water into a serving pitcher and discard the cooked lavender. Add the rest of the water, agave nectar, and lemon juice and stir well. Add the lavender sprigs and lemon slices and refrigerate until cool. Serve in slender, clear glasses.

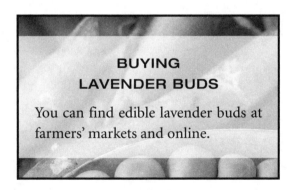

BUYING LAVENDER BUDS

You can find edible lavender buds at farmers' markets and online.

SPARKLING ROSEMARY LEMON-LIMEADE

Yield: 6 to 8 servings

Soundtrack: "I've Been in the Storm" by Fisk Jubilee Singers from *In Bright Mansions*

Fresh rosemary, which you can find at most supermarkets and farmers' markets, perfumes this lemon-limeade and gives it a medicinal twist. According to whole foods authority Rebecca Woods, rosemary is good for treating headaches, gas, and fevers.

---

2 cups water

6 fresh rosemary sprigs (2 to 3 inches each)

1/2 cup agave nectar or **Simple Syrup** (page 26)

6 tablespoons freshly squeezed lemon juice (from about 4 to 6 lemons)

6 tablespoons freshly squeezed lime juice (from about 6 to 8 limes)

4 cups sparkling water

1/2 large organic lime, ends cut off and sliced thinly lengthwise, for garnish

1/2 large organic lemon, ends cut off and sliced thinly lengthwise, for garnish

---

- In a small saucepan, combine 2 cups of water and 4 sprigs of rosemary, bring to a boil, and allow to boil vigorously, covered, for 10 minutes. Remove from heat and let steep for 10 minutes, then uncover and set aside to cool.

- Strain the rosemary water into a serving pitcher and compost the cooked rosemary sprigs. Add the agave nectar, lemon juice, and lime juice and stir well. Add the sparkling water and gently stir to combine. Add the remaining rosemary sprigs and the lemon/lime slices and refrigerate until cool. Serve in slender, clear glasses.

PURE STRAWBERRY POP

Yield: 2 servings

Soundtrack: "Green Corn" by Lead Belly from *Where Did You Sleep Last Night—Lead Belly Legacy, Vol. 1* and "Labels" by GZA from *Liquid Swords*

Film: *King Corn* (2007) by Ian Cheney and Curt Ellis. This informative and entertaining feature documentary captures two friends, one acre of corn, and the subsidized crop that drives our fast-food nation.

Full of artificial colors, flavors, sodium, caffeine, preservatives, and sugar, strawberry soda was one of my childhood favorites. Here is my version without all that "stuff" in it. It's simply fresh strawberries, agave nectar, and sparkling mineral water.

1 pint fresh strawberries, quartered

1 tablespoon agave nectar

2 cups sparkling mineral water

- Make strawberry nectar by combining the strawberries and agave nectar in an upright blender and pureeing until smooth, pushing down on the strawberries with a wooden spoon to ensure that they blend well. Strain the strawberry nectar through cheesecloth, to remove the tiny seeds, into a pitcher.
- Tilt the pitcher to one side, to minimize the amount of foam produced by the mineral water, and slowly pour in the water. *Gently* stir to mix the nectar and the water. Avoid over stirring to prevent the drink from foaming up too much and loosing its fizz.
- Serve over ice.

SOFT DRINKS

It's funny that the term "soft drink" is used to describe nonalcoholic, carbonated beverages because most are hard on your body. In case you don't already know, the majority of sodas include lots of caffeine, high-fructose corn syrup, denatured white sugar, preservatives, and artificial flavorings. And don't be fooled by a lot of those so-called commercial fruit juices. Unless it reads "100% Fruit Juice" on the bottle, your drink probably contains a small percentage of fruit juice and mostly sugars. Always read the labels.

SWEET, SOUR, AND SPICY BLACKBERRY LIMEADE

Yield: 6 to 8 servings

Soundtrack: "Unstoppable" by Santogold from *Santogold* and "Brooklyn Go Hard" by Jay-Z featuring Santogold from *Notorious*

This is a drink that I made while living in Brooklyn. It gave me a lot of comfort on those New-York-City-will-wear-you-out days. Remove the lime slices if storing in the refrigerator for more than a few hours, as they will make the drink bitter.

5 cups filtered water

½ cup agave nectar or **Simple Syrup** (page 26)

½ cup freshly squeezed lime juice (from about 10 to 12 limes)

⅛ teaspoon cayenne

About ½ pound (10 ounces) frozen blackberries

1 large organic lime, ends cut off and sliced thinly lengthwise

- In a large pitcher, combine the water, agave nectar, lime juice, and cayenne. Stir well. Add the blackberries and the lime slices, pour into a pitcher, and refrigerate until cool. Serve in slender, clear glasses.

PEOPLE'S PUNCH

Yield: 2 servings

Soundtrack: "My People" by Erykah Badu from *NuAmerykah Part One: The 4th World War,* "The People" by Common featuring Dwele from *Finding Forever,* "People" by J Dilla from *Donuts,* and "Pull Up the People" by M.I.A. from *Arular*

Book: *Race Rebels* by Robin D. G. Kelley (Fireside Press, 1996)

This is my nonalcoholic take on Planter's Punch, which usually contains rum. Dedicated to the people.

1 cup freshly squeezed orange juice

1/2 cup pomegranate juice

1/4 cup freshly squeezed lemon juice

1/4 cup freshly squeezed lime juice

2 tablespoons agave nectar

1 cup sparkling mineral water, chilled

2 organic orange slices, for garnish

- Combine the orange juice, pomegranate juice, lemon juice, lime juice, and agave nectar in a small pitcher and mix well. Serve in two ice-filled slender glasses, topping each glass off with 1/2 cup sparkling water and garnishing with orange slices.

SIN-GER [SIN JER] THIRST-QUENCHER

Yield: 12 to 14 servings

Soundtrack: "Souka Nayo" by Baaaba Maal from *Nomad Soul* and "Souka Nayo (Thievery Corporation Remix)" from *Afrikya, Vol. 1—A Musical Journey through Africa*

This drink is inspired by a tasty beverage served at Joloff, my favorite Senegalese restaurant in Brooklyn. They combine "sorrel" (a traditional Caribbean drink made from dried *Hibiscus sabdariffa*, commonly referred to as Jamaican or red sorrel) with a ginger drink to make their "Jolof Cocktail." You can buy dried "sorrel" in Caribbean and African specialty stores. Ask for dried hibiscus flowers if shopping elsewhere.

13 1/2 cups water

1 cup (about 1 ounce) dried hibiscus

1 cup fresh ginger juice (from 2 packed cups freshly grated ginger) (page 34)

1/4 cup fresh freshly squeezed lemon juice (about 3 to 4 lemons)

1 cup agave nectar or **Simple Syrup** (page 26)

- In a large saucepan over high heat, combine 7 cups water with the hibiscus. Bring to a boil. Reduce the heat and simmer, stirring occasionally, for 20 minutes. Remove from heat.
- Meanwhile, in a 1-gallon pitcher combine the ginger juice, lemon juice, agave nectar, and the remaining water and stir well. Refrigerate.
- Allow the hibiscus drink to cool for 2 hours and then strain into the pitcher with the ginger drink mixture. Mix well and refrigerate until cool.
- Serve over ice.

GINGER JUICE

To get ginger juice from ginger knobs, grate them on a coarse grater (no need to peel) or pulverize them in a food processor. Wrap them in cheese cloth and squeeze to extract all the juice. You can also squeeze the pulp through your hands without cheesecloth in batches and then strain the juice.

CINNAMON-APPLEJACK TODDY

Yield: 1 serving
Soundtrack: "Sanford and Son Theme (The Streetbeater)" by Quincy Jones from *20th Century Masters—The Millennium Collection: The Best of Quincy Jones*
Sitcom: *Sanford and Son* (seasons 1–4)
Book: *Revolution Televised* by Christine Acham (University of Minnesota Press, 2005)

In case you didn't know, *Sanford and Son* was *the* best American sitcom of the twentieth century (at least the first four out of six seasons). It is belly-achingly hilarious, slyly subversive, and brilliantly displays the many facets of African American humor. I grew up watching it with my Granny whenever I would sleep over at my paternal grandparents', and to this day I watch it several times a week (my parents bought me every season on DVD a few years ago). It is only fitting that I create a drink using Fred Sanford's alcoholic beverage of choice behind Ripple—applejack.

Applejack is an 80- to 100-proof American-made apple brandy that is aged for two years in wood. There are not many brands on the market, but Lairds Applejack is my brand of choice. This hot toddy is nice on a cold winter evening. It's warming, and "it'll make you sweat" (see episode seven from the first season of *Sanford and Son*).

1 cinnamon stick

3 tablespoons applejack (another brandy can be used in its place)

1 teaspoon apple juice

1 teaspoon freshly squeezed lemon juice

1 teaspoon agave nectar or 2 to 3
   Candied Orange Peels (page 189)

1 Granny Smith apple slice, for garnish

- Place the cinnamon stick at the bottom of a mug and add boiling water until the mug is a little over ½ full. Cover the mug with a plate and let it sit for 5 minutes. Add the applejack, apple juice, lemon juice, and agave nectar and gently stir until well combined; top off with more hot water. Add an apple slice to the mug and enjoy.

CALIFORNIA SLURRICANE

Yield: 2 servings
Soundtrack: "Big Chief" by Professor Longhair from *New Orleans Soul '60's*

In 2004 while living in Brooklyn and missing New Orleans, I created a **Frozen Blackberry Slurricane** (see *Grub*) in honor of the "Hurricane," a classic New Orleans cocktail. In 2006 while living in Oakland and missing Brooklyn and New Orleans, I created this drink. Next up: California Sake-cane.

½ cup light rum

½ cup dark rum

¼ cup freshly squeezed navel orange juice

½ cup freshly squeezed blood orange juice

2 tablespoons freshly squeezed lime juice

2 tablespoons pomegranate juice

2 tablespoons agave nectar or **Simple Syrup** (see page 26)

1 blood orange slice, for garnish

- Shake all the ingredients in a cocktail shaker with ice and strain into a hurricane (or comparable) glasses. Garnish with a blood orange slice.

FROZEN MEMPHIS MINT JULEP

Yield: 2 servings
Soundtrack: "Tennessee" by Arrested Development from *3 Years, 5 Months and 2 Days in the Life Of . . .* and "Alphabet Street" by Prince from *Lovesexy*

I used to wonder why some Southerners would make such a fuss over mint juleps. When I visited Louisville in 2007, around the time of the Kentucky Derby, I finally gave one a try. Now I know. A friend from Nashville asked me to create a version for "the ladies" so I came up with this one and gave it a Memphis twist. I replaced the bourbon with Jack Daniels, which has its distillery in Tennessee, and I added a touch of "Crown" to give it some Memphis crunk.

30 fresh mint leaves

4 teaspoons agave nectar

1/2 cup Jack Daniels

2 tablespoons Crown Royal

1 tablespoon water

12 ice cubes

2 long mint sprigs, for garnish

- Chill two pint-size canning jars in the freezer.
- To muddle the mint, combine the mint leaves and agave nectar at the bottom of a cup. Using the handle of a wooden spoon, crush the mint leaves until well pulverized, about 3 minutes.
- Add the Jack Daniels, Crown Royal, and water to the muddled mint and mix well. Transfer the mixture to an upright blender. Add the ice and blend until smooth, about 1 minute.
- Divide drink between two glasses and garnish each glass with a sprig of mint so your guests can get a whiff when they have a sip.

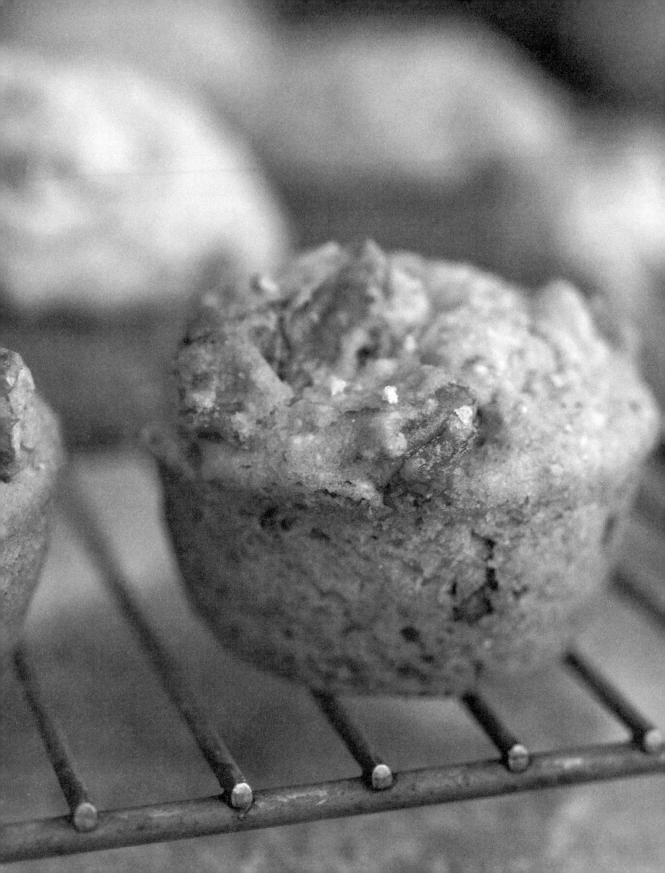

SOUND BITES
APPETIZERS. STARTERS. SNACKS.

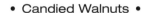

- Candied Walnuts •
• Double Maple-Coated Pecans •
• Spicy Goobers •
• Roasted Winter Squash Seeds •
• Minimalist Survival Snack Mix •

• Roasted Plantain Pieces with
Roasted Garlic–Lime Dipping Sauce •

• Crispy Okra Strips with Lime-Thyme Vinaigrette •

• Black-Eyed Pea Fritters with
Hot Pepper Sauce •

• Pan-Fried Coconut-Tempeh Cubes with
Creamy Celeriac Sauce •

• Baked Sweet Potato Fries with
Ginger-Peanut Dipping Sauce •

• Little Banana-Maple Pecan Cornbread Muffins •

• Garlicky Baby Lima Bean Spread •

• Some Things Are Small in Texas Caviar •

CANDIED WALNUTS

Yield: 4 cups

Soundtrack: "Bitter" by Me'Shell Ndegeocello from *Bitter*

Besides eating them as a snack, I use these often in green salads to add texture and sweetness.

---

4 cups raw walnut halves, toasted and skins removed (page 40)
1/4 cup extra-virgin olive oil
1/4 cup agave nectar
1/2 cup organic raw cane sugar

- In a large bowl, combine the walnuts with the olive oil and stir until thoroughly coated. Add the agave nectar and stir until thoroughly coated, then add the sugar and stir until thoroughly coated.

- Warm a large cast-iron skillet to medium-high. Add the walnuts, scraping the bowl to remove everything, and stir constantly until the walnuts are fragrant and most of the liquid has evaporated, about 1 1/2 minutes.

- Transfer the walnuts to parchment paper and quickly spread out, separating them with two forks. Set aside to cool.

TOASTING WALNUTS AND REMOVING THEIR SKINS

While naturally sweet in flavor, walnuts have a bitter outer skin. So right before using them I remove it. First, preheat the oven to 350°F. Spread the walnuts on a large baking sheet and toast for 8 minutes, stirring halfway through the cooking. Remove from oven to cool. Transfer walnuts to a sieve and, holding the sieve over the sink, rub the walnuts against the wire until the skins loosen and fall off. Set aside to completely cool. While you will get the freshest most flavorful walnuts by purchasing them in the shell and cracking them before using, it can be time consuming. So I buy shelled, whole walnut halves and store them in the freezer.

DOUBLE MAPLE-COATED PECANS

Yield: 4 cups

Soundtrack: "Hunter" by Björk from *Homogenic*

Since Paw-Paw, my paternal grandfather, had a gigantic pecan tree in his front yard, those oblong nuts were the cheapest snack for my cousins and me to get our hands on back in the day, so we went foraging daily. I love to eat them plain, but this version, coated with maple syrup and maple sugar, makes a nice after-dinner treat to satisfy my sweet tooth. Since shelled pecans have a shorter shelf life than most nuts, I always store them in the freezer.

4 cups raw pecan halves

1/4 cup extra-virgin olive oil

1/4 cup pure maple syrup

1/2 cup maple sugar (you can also use organic raw cane sugar)

- Preheat the oven to 350°F.
- Spread the pecans on a large baking sheet and toast for 4 minutes, stirring halfway through the cooking.
- Remove the pecans to a large bowl, add the olive oil, and stir with a wooden spoon until thoroughly coated. Add the maple syrup and stir until thoroughly coated. Then add the maple sugar and stir until thoroughly coated.
- Warm a large cast-iron skillet to medium-high. Add the pecans, scraping the bowl to remove everything, and stir constantly with a wooden spoon until pecans are fragrant and most of the liquid has evaporated, about 2 1/2 to 3 minutes.
- Transfer the pecans to parchment paper and quickly spread out, separating them with two forks. Set aside to cool.
- Serve warm.

LIGHTLY TOASTING NUTS AND SEEDS

Toasted nuts and seeds add texture, unique flavors, and a touch of protein to salads, stir-fries, and other dishes. To bring out their natural oil and enhance the taste of nuts and seeds, toast them in a dry skillet over medium heat, shaking often, until fragrant, about 4 minutes; or toast on a baking sheet in an oven at 325°F for 5 to 7 minutes, shaking the pan a few times for even cooking. Nuts and seeds contain oils that will go rancid, so I store mine in the freezer.

SPICY GOOBERS

Yield: 4 cups

Soundtrack: "Salt Peanuts" by Charlie "Bird" Parker from *The Complete Live Performances on Savoy*, "Salt Peanuts" by Dizzy Gillespie from *Salt Peanuts*, "Salt Peanuts" by Miles Davis Quintet from *Steamin'*, and "Salt Peanuts" by Bud Powell from *The Lonely One*

Art: "Horn Players" by Jean-Michel Basquiat

No. These aren't chocolate-covered peanuts. Derived from the African Bantu word "nguba," the word "goober" was commonly used in the South to refer to peanuts a few generations ago. While I like starting from scratch, using raw peanuts for this dish, you can use preroasted and go right to the third step in this recipe (omit the salt in the spice mixture if the ones you use are salted). I highly recommend purchasing organic peanuts, as their conventional counterparts tend to be heavily treated with chemicals.

I dedicate this zesty snack to my folks at Farmer Brown Restaurant in San Francisco, where they serve a similar treat at the bar during happy hour.

And big up to the late George Washington Carver.

---

4 cups raw shelled peanuts
2 teaspoons onion powder
1 teaspoon garlic powder
2 teaspoons paprika
2 teaspoons chili powder
¼ teaspoon cayenne
1 teaspoon organic raw cane sugar
1 teaspoon fine sea salt
3 tablespoons peanut oil

- Preheat the oven to 350°F.
- Spread nuts in an even layer on a parchment-lined baking sheet. Bake, stirring every 5 minutes to ensure even roasting, until starting to crisp and fragrant, about 20 minutes.
- While the peanuts are roasting, combine the onion powder, garlic powder, paprika, chili powder, cayenne, sugar, and salt in a small bowl and mix well. Set aside.
- Add the peanut oil to a large bowl. Transfer the roasted peanuts to the bowl and stir well to coat. Add the spice blend to the bowl and stir well to coat. Transfer the peanuts back to the baking sheet and roast for 5 more minutes.
- Remove from oven and cool for 15 minutes before eating.
- Store in an airtight container in the refrigerator.

ROASTED WINTER SQUASH SEEDS

Yield: how ever many seeds you get from your squash
Soundtrack: "Squash All Beef" by KRS-One from *KRS-One*
Book: *Bullsh*t or Fertilizer* by Pierre Bennu (Andrews McMeel Publishing, 2003)

The next time a recipe calls for a winter squash (or watermelon) DON'T THROW AWAY THE SEEDS. They can be roasted and eaten as a tasty snack or used as a garnish for **Butternut Squash–Bartlett Pear Soup with Roasted Butternut Squash Seeds** (page 80). It's kinda hard to write this recipe since you never know how many seeds a given squash will yield. I usually add enough oil to lightly coat the seeds, toss them with dried spices such as salt, black pepper, and paprika, and then roast them until golden brown. Use this recipe as a guide and adjust it to suit the amount of seeds you scrape from your squash.

1/2 cup winter squash seeds
1 teaspoon extra-virgin olive oil
1/4 teaspoon coarse sea salt
1/8 teaspoon paprika
1/8 teaspoon black pepper

- Preheat the oven to 275°F.
- Line a baking sheet with parchment paper.
- After removing the seeds from the squash, you can rinse them with cold water, and remove any squash remnants (although I leave that stuff on the seeds). Pat dry with a clean towel or paper towel and transfer to a small bowl. Add the olive oil and toss well until evenly coated. Next add the salt, paprika, and pepper and toss until evenly coated. Spread out in an even layer on the prepared baking sheet.
- Bake, stirring every 5 minutes, until lightly browned, about 15 minutes.
- Remove from the oven and cool before serving.

MINIMALIST SURVIVAL SNACK MIX

Yield: 3½ cups
Soundtrack: "Runaway Slave" by
Showbiz & A. G. from *Runaway Slave*

With snack mix it's all about balance—
sweet/salty, chewy/crunchy, fruity/nutty—
and this simple mix maintains perfect
equilibrium in all areas. I actually created
this recipe running out of my house on the
way to the airport for a six-hour flight. I
wanted something light to quell any
hunger pangs, so I dumped some recently
toasted walnuts into a resealable plastic bag
full of raisins. The earthiness of the walnuts and the sugariness of the raisins com-
pliment each other well.

2 cups raw walnut halves, toasted
(page 40)
1½ cups Thompson raisins

- In a container that can be sealed tightly,
mix the walnuts with the raisins and shake
until well combined.

ROASTED PLANTAIN PIECES WITH ROASTED GARLIC–LIME DIPPING SAUCE

Yield: 4 to 6 servings

Soundtrack: "Justicia" by Eddie Palmieri from *Fania Live 03 from San Francisco DJ Sake One*

I originally roasted plantain pieces to add to my **Upper Caribbean Creamy Grits with Roasted Plantains Pieces** (page 135) and give that dish some texture. When I first tested that recipe, the plantains I used were slightly yellow—almost green—and reminded me of the flavor of *tostones* (twice-fried plantains found in Latin American cuisine). So I decided that I would pair them with garlic dipping sauce to make a tasty appetizer. According to Raúl Musibay, Cuban cookbook author and cofounder of icuban.com, tostones can be linked directly to the African continent: "The tradition of the tostone comes from African slaves. In the Congo, the people prepare plantains in the exact same way, even to this day."

Roasted Garlic–Lime Dipping Sauce

All the cloves from one head of roasted garlic (page 77)
1/4 cup extra-virgin olive oil
1 tablespoon minced cilantro
1/4 cup freshly squeezed lime juice
1/4 cup water
1/4 teaspoon coarse sea salt
Freshly ground white pepper

Roasted Plantains

3 large, slightly ripe yellow plantains, ends cut off, peeled, cut in half lengthwise and cut into 1/2-inch pieces widthwise
1 tablespoon extra-virgin olive oil

For the dipping sauce

- In an upright blender, combine the roasted garlic, olive oil, cilantro, lime juice, water, and 1/4 teaspoon salt. Puree until creamy. Season with white pepper and salt to taste.

For the plantains

- Preheat oven to 450°F.
- In a small bowl, toss the plantains and the olive oil. Transfer to a parchment-lined baking sheet and cook, stirring a few times to ensure even browning, until crisp on the outside and starting to turn golden brown, about 30 minutes.
- Transfer the plantain pieces to a serving platter and scatter them around the dipping sauce. Have toothpicks handy for easy dipping.

CRISPY OKRA STRIPS WITH LIME-THYME VINAIGRETTE

Yield: 4 to 6 servings
Soundtrack: "Okra" by Olu Dara from
In the World—From Natchez to New York

To be honest, there are only a few ways that I like to have okra, as I generally find it to be too slimy for my taste. This is one of them.

---

1 pound small to medium okra pods, ends cut off and quartered lengthwise

1/2 cup **Multipurpose Coating for Dredging Foods** (page 167)

3 tablespoons freshly squeezed lime juice

1 teaspoon red wine vinegar

1 teaspoon Dijon mustard

1 small clove garlic, minced

1 tablespoon fresh thyme, minced

1/2 teaspoon coarse sea salt

8 tablespoons extra-virgin olive oil

White pepper

- In a large bowl, cover the okra strips with cold water, refrigerate, and soak for 15 minutes.
- Transfer the strips to a colander and rinse well under cold running water for 2 to 3 minutes.
- Put the strips back in the bowl, cover with water, and refrigerate for an additional 15 minutes.
- Transfer the okra back to the colander, rinse well under cold running water for 2 to 3 minutes, and let drain. With paper towels or a clean kitchen towel, pat the okra strips as much as possible to dry them (they will be slightly moist).
- In a medium-size bowl, combine the okra strips with the Multipurpose Coating for Dredging Foods and toss them around to coat well.

- Make the vinaigrette by combining the lime juice, vinegar, mustard, garlic, thyme, and salt in an upright blender. Blend while slowly pouring in the olive oil. Add white pepper to taste.
- In a large, nonstick skillet over medium-high heat, warm the vinaigrette, just until it starts to bubble. Pour in the okra mixture and let it cook for 4 to 5 minutes, until it begins to brown (the pieces will start forming cakes). With a wooden spatula, turn over the pieces and cook for another 4 to 5 minutes, until browning and crisp.
- Transfer the okra to a paper towel–lined baking sheet to drain. Then arrange on a platter and serve hot.

OKRA

Also know as ladyfingers and gumbo, okra originated in what is now Ethiopia over ten thousand years ago and is used in African, Afro-Caribbean, and African American cuisine. In addition to being served sautéed, grilled, or pickled, it is often used as a thickener in stews and gumbos. Select smaller okra pods, as they are more tender and less slimy than bigger ones. If you can find it, try purple okra.

BLACK-EYED PEA FRITTERS WITH HOT PEPPER SAUCE

Yield: 4 to 6 servings

Soundtrack: "I.T.T., Pt. 2" by Fela Kuti from *The Best Best of Fela Kuti*

Art: "Three Wise Men Greeting Entry into Lagos" by Kehinde Wiley

Books: *How Europe Underdeveloped Africa* by Walter Rodney (Howard University Press, 1981) and *Graceland* by Chris Abani (Picador, 2005)

While bean fritters are thought to have their origin in Nigeria, one can find them throughout West Africa. Inspired by the Black-Eyed Pea Fritters served at the Gambian-Cameroonian restaurant Bennachin in New Orleans, I whipped up this dish.

1 cup dried black-eyed peas, sorted, soaked overnight, drained, and rinsed

1/2 medium onion, diced

1/2 cup raw peanuts

1 teaspoon minced thyme

1/4 teaspoon cayenne

1 tablespoon apple cider vinegar

1/4 cup plus 2 tablespoons water

1 teaspoon coarse sea salt

1/2 cup finely chopped green bell pepper

1 tablespoon cornmeal

5 cups coconut oil

- Remove the skins from the beans by adding them to a large bowl, filling the bowl with water, agitating the beans, and fishing out the skins that float to the top with a fine mesh strainer. Rinse beans well.
- In a food processor fitted with a metal blade, combine the beans, onion, peanuts, thyme, cayenne, vinegar, water, and salt and pulse until completely smooth. Transfer to a medium bowl, cover, and refrigerate for 1 hour.
- Preheat the oven to 200°F.
- Remove the batter from the refrigerator, add the bell pepper and cornmeal, and beat with a wooden spoon for 2 minutes.
- In a medium-size saucepan over high heat, warm the coconut oil until hot but not smoking, about 5 minutes.

- Lower the oil to medium high, and in batches of 5, spoon the batter into the oil, 1 tablespoon at a time. Fry, stirring around, until golden brown, about 2 minutes. If necessary, adjust the temperature to ensure that the fritters do not cook too quickly.

- Transfer the fritters to a paper towel–lined plate and allow them to drain. Transfer the drained fritters to a baking sheet and place in the oven to keep warm.
- Serve hot with **Hot Pepper Sauce** (page 171).

BLACK-EYED PEAS

African in origin, black-eyed peas are one of the most salient staples of African American cooking. They tend to cook quickly, but if they are old, it may take longer to prepare them. While canned black-eyed peas are available, I always make mine from scratch. In Southern lore black-eyed peas are thought to bring good luck when eaten in copious amounts on New Year's Day. So my family slow-cooks them in a Crock-Pot every December 31.

PAN-FRIED COCONUT-TEMPEH CUBES WITH CREAMY CELERIAC SAUCE

Yield: 6 to 8 servings

Soundtrack: "Dollar" by Steve Spacek from *Space Shift*

I created this dish as an ode to the breaded fried shrimp served with ré-moulade, a creamy dip eaten with seafood, that I used to enjoy when my family visited New Orleans.

1 cup coconut oil

1 pound (2 8-ounce packages) tempeh cut into 1/2-inch cubes

Fine sea salt

1 cup **Creamy Celeriac Sauce** (page 170)

- In a large sauté pan over medium heat, warm the coconut oil until hot but not smoking. Fry the tempeh in batches until golden brown, about 2 1/2 minutes each side. Transfer to a paper towel–lined plate and *immediately* sprinkle with salt so the tempeh can absorb it.

- Transfer the tempeh cubes to a serving platter and scatter them around a bowl full of sauce. Have toothpicks handy for easy dipping.

BAKED SWEET POTATO FRIES WITH GINGER-PEANUT DIPPING SAUCE

Yield: 4 servings

Soundtrack: "Oppression" by Ben Harper from *Fight for Your Mind*

This is a healthier and sweeter alternative to fried white potatoes. But if you want to indulge occasionally, feel free to deep-fry these in organic, unrefined coconut oil until lightly browned, 3 to 4 minutes.

Fries

4 uniformly shaped medium sweet potatoes (about 2 pounds), peeled

1 teaspoon coarse sea salt

1 tablespoon extra-virgin olive oil

Dipping Sauce

1 heaping tablespoon minced ginger

1/2 cup toasted peanuts (page 41)

1/2 cup apple juice

1 teaspoon agave nectar

1/8 teaspoon cayenne

1/4 teaspoon coarse sea salt

For the fries

- Cut the potatoes into slices about 1/2-inch thick and then cut them 1/2-inch lengthwise into the shape of fries.
- Preheat the oven to 450°F.
- Combine the sweet potatoes, 3 quarts cold water, and 1 teaspoon salt in a large pot over high heat. Parboil, uncovered, for 10 minutes. Drain in a colander and pat well with a clean kitchen towel or paper towels until *completely dry*.
- In a large bowl, toss the sweet potatoes with the olive oil.
- Arrange fries on a parchment-lined baking sheet and bake for 50 minutes, gently stirring every 15 minutes with a wooden spoon to ensure even browning, until tender and caramelized.

For the dipping sauce

- In an upright blender, combine the ginger, peanuts, apple juice, agave nectar, cayenne, and salt and blend until creamy. Transfer to a small serving bowl.

LITTLE BANANA-MAPLE PECAN CORNBREAD MUFFINS

Yield: about 24 mini-muffins
Soundtrack: "Angel" by Massive Attack from *Mezzanine,* "A.N.G.E.L." (Reprise)" by Dwele from *Subject,* and "Angel" by Anita Baker from *The Songstress*

These delicious muffins are not quite a dessert but I feel like I'm indulging when I eat them. Banana imparts a light, sugary taste that complements the earthy-sweet flavor of the **Double-Maple Coated Pecans** (page 41) well. The cornmeal (along with the pecans) creates a satisfying, crunchy texture. A cold glass of **Almond Milk** (page 28) makes a delicious accompaniment for these treats.

---

3 tablespoons unrefined corn oil plus
   more for greasing the tin
1¼ cups yellow cornmeal
½ cup all-purpose flour
¼ cup whole wheat pastry flour
2 tablespoons organic raw cane sugar
1 teaspoon baking powder
1 teaspoon baking soda
¾ teaspoon fine sea salt
1 large ripe banana
1 cup unflavored rice milk
2 tablespoons pure maple syrup
¾ cup **Double Maple-Coated**
   Pecans (page 41), chopped

- Set a rack in the middle of the oven and preheat the oven to 425°F.
- Grease a mini-muffin tin with corn oil and set aside.
- In a large bowl, whisk together the cornmeal, flours, sugar, baking powder, baking soda, and salt.
- In an upright blender, combine the banana, rice milk, maple syrup, and the remaining corn oil, and blend until creamy.
- Transfer the muffin tin to the oven to preheat for 5 minutes, until sizzling.
- In the last minute of the muffin tin preheating, combine the wet mixture with the dry mixture by mixing with a spoon just until blended, being careful not to overmix. Fold in the nuts.
- Remove the tin from the oven and spoon the batter into the muffin slots until they are three-quarters full. Return to the oven and bake on the center rack for 13 to 15 minutes, until the tops are golden.
- Serve immediately.

GARLICKY BABY LIMA BEAN SPREAD

Yield: 4 to 6 servings

Soundtrack: "Lima Beans" by Algia Mae Hinton from *Honey Babe*

I love the sweet flavor of fresh lima beans, and they are perfect for making **Succotash Soup with Garlicky Cornbread Croutons** (page 88). But the denser, starchier flavor of dried limas makes them better suited for this spread that I serve with crudités, crackers, or toasted bread.

- -

1 cup dried baby lima beans, sorted, soaked overnight, drained, and rinsed

1 3-inch piece kombu

1/4 teaspoon coarse sea salt

1 tablespoon extra-virgin olive oil plus more for drizzling

5 cloves garlic, minced

1 teaspoon ground cumin

1/4 teaspoon red pepper flakes

1 teaspoon minced fresh sage

2 tablespoons freshly squeezed lemon juice

1 teaspoon finely grated lemon zest

1/4 teaspoon freshly ground white pepper

- -

- In a medium-size saucepan over high heat, combine the lima beans and the kombu with enough water to cover by 1 inch and bring to a boil. Skim off any foam, reduce the heat to medium, and simmer, partially covered, for 45 minutes. Add 1 teaspoon salt and simmer for another 15 minutes. Drain the beans. Remove the kombu and compost it.

- While the beans are cooking, in a small sauté pan, combine 1 tablespoon of the olive oil with the garlic, cumin, and red pepper flakes over medium heat. Sauté for 1 1/2 minutes, until fragrant, then add the sage and 1/4 teaspoon salt. Sauté for another 30 seconds then remove from heat.

- To make the dip, combine the beans, sautéed garlic mixture, lemon juice, lemon zest, 1/4 teaspoon salt, and 1/4 teaspoon white pepper in a food processor fitted with a metal blade. Process until smooth. Transfer to a serving bowl and drizzle with olive oil.

SOME THINGS ARE SMALL IN TEXAS CAVIAR

Yield: 4 to 6 servings

Soundtrack: "One Day" by UGK from *Ridin' Dirty*

Don't worry—this dish does not contain fish eggs. Texas Caviar is simply another creative way that someone conjured up to prepare black-eyed peas. My version uses sun-dried tomatoes to give the salad a sweet and intense flavor. It can be served cold or at room temperature, and it makes a tasty appetizer along with grilled or toasted bread. If you can't find unsalted sun-dried tomatoes simply omit the salt in the recipe.

1 cup oil-packed sun-dried tomatoes (unsalted)

1 cup dried black-eyed peas, sorted, soaked overnight, drained, and rinsed

1 3-inch piece kombu

Coarse sea salt

3 tablespoons freshly squeezed lemon juice

2 tablespoons red wine vinegar

2 cloves garlic, minced

1/4 cup extra-virgin olive oil

1 serrano chile, sliced thinly

1 cup finely diced celery

1/2 cup finely diced green bell pepper

1/2 cup finely diced red bell pepper

1/2 cup minced fresh parsley

Freshly ground white pepper

- Put the tomatoes in a bowl. Add enough boiling water to cover them and set aside for 20 minutes.

- Meanwhile get the beans started. In a medium saucepan over high heat, combine the black-eyed peas and kombu with enough water to cover by 2 inches and bring to a boil. Skim off any foam, reduce the heat to medium, and simmer, partially covered, for 50 minutes. Add 2 teaspoons salt and simmer for another 10 minutes, until softened but still firm. Drain the beans, rinse in cold water for a minute or so, and set aside to cool. Remove the kombu and compost it.

- Drain the tomatoes, reserving the cooking liquid, and transfer to an upright blender.
- Add the lemon juice, vinegar, garlic, olive oil, chile, 1/4 teaspoon salt, 3 tablespoons of the reserved tomato cooking liquid, and the reconstituted tomatoes to the blender and blend until creamy.
- In a large bowl, combine the celery, green and red bell pepper, parsley, the beans, and 1/2 cup of the tomato dressing (save the rest to be used as a spread or something) and mix with a spoon until well coated. Refrigerate until ready to serve.
- Remove from the refrigerator 30 minutes before serving to bring up to room temperature. Season with salt and pepper to taste before serving.

KOMBU

Kombu is a sea vegetable that enhances the flavor (and nutrients) of beans and makes them more digestible. I usually remove mine before serving as I would a bay leaf. You can buy dried kombu at Asian markets and natural food stores, and you can order it online.

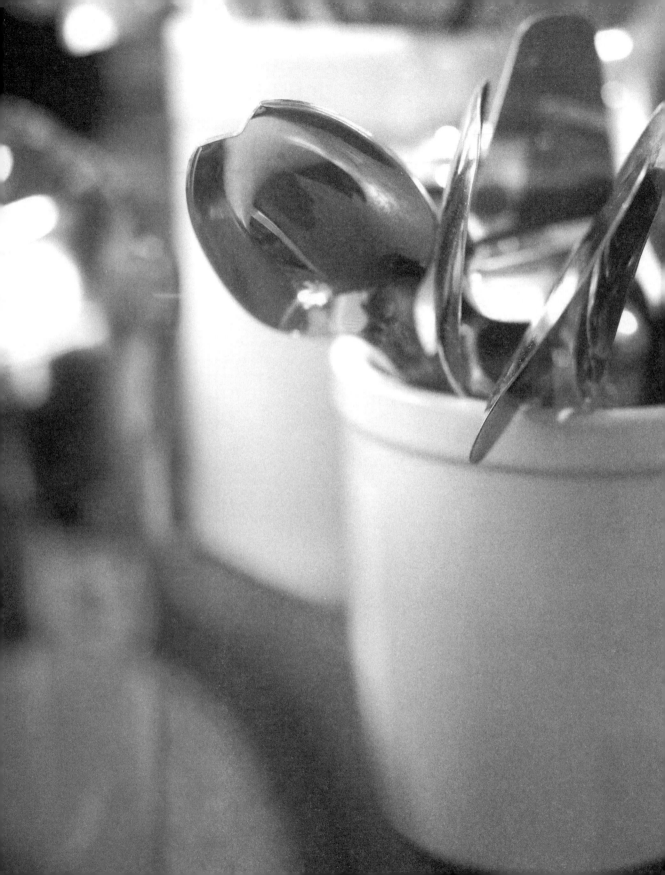

MIX PLATES
SALADS. SLAWS. DRESSINGS.

• Basic Vinaigrette •

• Garlicky Creamy Vinaigrette •

• Shredded Beet, Apple, and
Currant Salad with Apple Vinaigrette •

• Shaved Cucumber Salad with Citrus-Cilantro Dressing •

• Straightforward Coleslaw •

• Carrot-Cayenne Coleslaw •

• Carrot-Cranberry-Walnut Salad with
Creamy Walnut Vinaigrette •

• Chilled Citrus-Broccoli Salad •

• Roasted Red Potato Salad with
Parsley–Pine Nut Pesto •

• Chilled and Grilled Okra, Corn, and
Heirloom Tomato Salad •

• Wild Style Salad (Rock the Bells Remix) •

• Caramelized Grapefruit, Avocado,
and Watercress Salad with Grapefruit Vinaigrette •

BASIC VINAIGRETTE

Yield: about ¾ cup
Soundtrack: "Can It All Be So Simple"
by Wu-Tang Clan from *Enter the Wu-Tang*
(36 Chambers)

This light, all-purpose vinaigrette is great
for dressing simple lettuce salads and
steamed vegetables.

2 tablespoons freshly squeezed
   lemon juice
1 tablespoon red wine vinegar
¼ teaspoon Dijon mustard
1 large clove garlic, minced
Coarse sea salt
½ cup extra-virgin olive oil
Freshly ground white pepper

- In an upright blender, combine the lemon juice, vinegar, mustard, garlic, and ½ teaspoon salt. Blend while slowly pouring in the olive oil. Season with salt and pepper to taste.

GARLICKY CREAMY VINAIGRETTE

Yield: about ¾ cup
Soundtrack: "C.R.E.A.M." by
Wu-Tang Clan from *Enter the Wu-Tang*
(36 Chambers)

This is a standard vinaigrette with silken tofu added for creaminess and garlic added for punch. In addition to dressing lettuce salads and steamed vegetables, I sometimes drizzle this dressing on fresh heirloom tomatoes.

2 tablespoons freshly squeezed
    lemon juice

2 tablespoons apple cider vinegar

1 teaspoon Dijon mustard

2 large cloves garlic, minced

1 tablespoon chopped fresh herbs such
    as tarragon, basil, parsley, or thyme

Coarse sea salt

¼ cup silken tofu

2 tablespoons extra-virgin olive oil

Freshly ground white pepper

- In an upright blender, combine the lemon juice, vinegar, mustard, garlic, herbs, ½ teaspoon salt, and tofu. Blend while slowly adding the olive oil. Season with salt and pepper to taste.

MAKING SALAD DRESSINGS AND DRESSING SALADS

Although I suggest using an upright blender for making all of the vinaigrettes in this book, you can actually whisk most of them in a bowl. I just prefer the creaminess of blended salad dressings (plus I'm lazy). In terms of dressing your salads, do so immediately before serving. And be sure not to overdress them or the dressing will overpower the flavor of your greens and quickly make them limp. Use just enough to lightly coat them.

SHREDDED BEET, APPLE, AND CURRANT SALAD WITH APPLE VINAIGRETTE

Yield: 4 to 6 servings
Soundtrack: "Boom" by
Georgia Anne Muldrow from *Olesi:
Fragments of an Earth*

Sometimes I make salad buffets when
I'm having friends over during the summer. This one is usually the brightest and
sweetest on the table.

2 large fresh beets, peeled, roots
   trimmed, and coarsely grated
2 large firm apples, such as Rome,
   Crispin, or Granny Smith, cored,
   peeled, and coarsely grated
2 cups apple juice
2 teaspoons apple cider vinegar
1/4 teaspoon coarse sea salt
2 tablespoons extra-virgin olive oil
Freshly ground white pepper
1/2 cup currants

- Combine the shredded beets and apples
  in a large bowl.
- Meanwhile, in a small saucepan over high
  heat, bring the apple juice to a boil and reduce the juice to a little less than 1/2 cup,
  about 15 minutes. Transfer 1 tablespoon
  of the reduced apple juice to an upright
  blender (reserve the rest for another dish
  or dilute with water and drink).
- Make the vinaigrette by adding the apple
  cider vinegar and salt to the blender and
  blending while slowly pouring in the olive
  oil. Season with white pepper to taste.
- Add currants and the dressing to the bowl
  with the beets and apples and massage
  with clean hands until well dressed, 3 to 5
  minutes.

SHAVED CUCUMBER SALAD WITH CITRUS-CILANTRO DRESSING

Yield: 4 to 6 servings
Soundtrack: "Chill Out" by Black Uhuru from *Liberation—The Island Anthology*

This is a simple, cooling salad that can be enjoyed for a light lunch on summer days or as a side to a heavier entrée.

6 medium cucumbers, peeled

1 teaspoon coarse sea salt

2 tablespoons freshly squeezed orange juice

1 tablespoon freshly squeezed lemon juice

1 tablespoon freshly squeezed lime juice

1/4 cup minced fresh cilantro

1 teaspoon agave nectar

Freshly ground white pepper

- With a Y-shaped peeler cut thin strips from the cucumbers, stopping when you get to the seeds (compost the core), and transfer the strips to a medium bowl. Toss the cucumbers with the salt. Refrigerate for 20 minutes.

- In another bowl, combine the orange juice, lemon juice, lime juice, cilantro, agave nectar, and white pepper to taste. Whisk well to combine. Set aside.

- Drain the cucumbers and transfer them to the bowl with the dressing. Toss well to combine. Cover and refrigerate for at least 30 minutes, tossing every 10 minutes. With a slotted spoon, transfer the cucumbers to a salad bowl and serve.

STRAIGHTFORWARD COLESLAW

Yield: 4 to 6 servings
Soundtrack: "Think" by Aretha Franklin from *Aretha Now*

Coleslaw is always present at my family's summer gatherings. So I created this easy-to-make version to dissuade folks from buying the prepackaged mixes that suggest that you add tons of mayonnaise. Once the vinaigrette is made for this one, you can pass it over to the kiddies to massage into the cabbage (with thoroughly clean hands of course).

1 small green cabbage head, cored, quartered, and sliced thinly
1/2 teaspoon Dijon mustard
1/4 cup silken tofu
2 tablespoons red wine vinegar
1 teaspoon agave nectar
1 teaspoon coarse sea salt
2 tablespoons extra-virgin olive oil

- Place the green cabbage in a large bowl.
- In an upright blender, combine the mustard, tofu, vinegar, agave nectar, and salt. While blending, slowly add the olive oil.
- Add the dressing to the green cabbage and massage until it shrinks down, about 3 to 4 minutes. Cover, and refrigerate for at least 1 hour and remove at least 15 minutes before serving.

CARROT-CAYENNE COLESLAW

Yield: 4 to 6 servings
Soundtrack: "Happy Talk" by Nancy Wilson and Cannonball Adderley from *Nancy Wilson & Cannonball Adderley*

This version is equally simple to make, but it is more visually stimulating and has a kick that comes from the cayenne.

1/2 small green cabbage head, cored and sliced thinly

2 large carrots, grated

1/4 small purple cabbage head, cored and sliced thinly

1/2 teaspoon Dijon mustard

1/4 cup champagne vinegar

1 teaspoon agave nectar or organic raw cane sugar

1 teaspoon coarse sea salt

1/4 teaspoon cayenne

3 tablespoons extra-virgin olive oil

2 tablespoons sesame seeds, toasted

- Place the green cabbage and carrots in one bowl and the purple cabbage in a separate bowl.
- In an upright blender, combine the mustard, vinegar, agave nectar, salt, and cayenne. While blending, slowly add the olive oil.
- Add half of the dressing to the green cabbage/carrots and add the remaining dressing to the purple cabbage. Massage them both well until wilted, about 3 to 5 minutes each. Cover, and refrigerate them for at least 1 hour or overnight. Remove at least 15 minutes before serving, combine them, add the sesame seeds, and mix well.

CARROT-CRANBERRY-WALNUT SALAD WITH CREAMY WALNUT VINAIGRETTE

Yield: 4 to 6 servings

Soundtrack: "Too Tough to Die" by Martina Topley-Bird from *Anything*

This is a modern spin on my mom's carrot-raisin salad. Rather than adding dollops of mayonnaise to the dish, I combine silken tofu with the vinaigrette to make it creamier and use tangy dried cranberries instead of raisins. The walnuts add texture to the salad and give it a more robust flavor.

Dressing

- 1 tablespoon freshly squeezed lemon juice
- 2 tablespoons apple cider vinegar
- 1 tablespoon Dijon mustard
- 1/4 cup silken tofu
- 1/2 teaspoon coarse sea salt
- 2 tablespoons walnut oil

Salad

- 3 cups coarsely grated carrots (5–6 large carrots)
- 1/4 cup dried cranberries
- 1 cup walnuts, toasted and skins removed (page 40)

- In a blender, combine the lemon juice, vinegar, mustard, tofu, and salt. Blend while slowly pouring in the walnut oil.
- In a large bowl, combine the carrots, cranberries, and vinaigrette. With clean hands, toss the salad well, thoroughly coating it with the vinaigrette. Cover and chill for at least 30 minutes. Remove from the refrigerator 10 minutes before serving, add the walnuts, and toss well.

CHILLED CITRUS-BROCCOLI SALAD

Yield: 4 to 6 servings
Soundtrack: "Bossa Per Due (Thievery Corporation Remix)" by Nicola Conte from *Jet Sounds Revisited*

If you're looking for a nutrient-dense vegetable to help you load up on vitamin C (twice as much as an orange), calcium (as much as milk), and other antioxidants, make sure you eat your broccoli. This salad is a good place to start getting your fill. Once I made it for a group of kids, and they were begging for seconds. Seriously. While most people only eat the head of broccoli, I suggest including the equally nutritious stalk as well. But make sure you peel it first.

2½ teaspoons coarse sea salt

2 large heads broccoli, florets separated, stalks peeled and sliced thinly

1 tablespoon freshly squeezed orange juice

1 tablespoon freshly squeezed lime juice

2 tablespoons freshly squeezed lemon juice

1 tablespoon agave nectar

1 teaspoon chopped fresh basil

3 cloves garlic, minced

9 tablespoons extra-virgin olive oil

- In a large pot over high heat, bring 3 quarts of water to a boil, add 2 teaspoons of salt, and dissolve. Remove pot from heat, add the broccoli for one minute, until bright green, and drain.
- In a blender, make the marinade by combining the orange juice, lime juice, lemon juice, agave nectar, basil, garlic, and ½ teaspoon salt. Blend while slowly pouring in the olive oil.
- Place the broccoli in a large bowl and add the marinade. With clean hands, massage the broccoli for 3 to 5 minutes, thoroughly coating it with the marinade. Cover and chill for at least 30 minutes, or overnight.
- Serve cold.

ROASTED RED POTATO SALAD WITH PARSLEY–PINE NUT PESTO

Yield: 6 to 8 servings

Soundtrack: "Friends" by Ann Peebles and Don Bryant from *Fill This World with Love*

My family usually serves run-of-the-mill, drowned-in-mayonnaise potato salad at cookouts, so I knew that I had to provide an equally satisfying alternative to mix it up a little bit. This is it. The vibrant pesto deepens the flavor of the potatoes and the roasted peppers provide sweet bursts with every bite. Once, I brought this version to a family reunion and it was gone before I could get any. I didn't even trip.

Pesto

- ⅓ cup pine nuts
- 2 cups loosely packed, flat-leaf parsley leaves
- 2 medium cloves garlic, peeled
- 1 tablespoon mellow white or yellow miso
- ¼ cup freshly squeezed lemon juice
- ½ cup extra-virgin olive oil
- ½ teaspoon coarse sea salt

Salad

- 2 pounds small red potatoes, cut into 1-inch chunks
- 1 tablespoon extra-virgin olive oil
- 3 large red bell peppers, seeded and cut into 1-inch dice
- Coarse sea salt
- Freshly ground white pepper

For the pesto

- Preheat the oven to 350°F.
- Arrange the pine nuts on a baking sheet and toast them for about 8 minutes, stirring after 4 minutes.
- In the bowl of a food processor fitted with a metal blade, combine the pine nuts, parsley, garlic, miso, and lemon juice and puree. Slowly add the olive oil and process until smooth. Add ½ teaspoon salt and set aside.

For the salad

- Preheat the oven to 400°F.
- In a large bowl, combine the potatoes and the olive oil. Toss to coat. Transfer the potatoes to a parchment-lined rimmed baking sheet and roast for 20 minutes, stirring after 10 minutes. Add the bell peppers to the baking sheet and stir to combine. Roast for 1 hour, stirring every 15 minutes, until the potatoes are tender and the bell peppers well roasted.

- Transfer the potatoes and bell peppers to a large bowl, add 1/2 cup plus 3 tablespoons of pesto (or more if you want it creamier), stir well, and season with salt and pepper to taste. Serve at room temperature. Cover the remaining pesto with a film of olive oil in a tightly sealed jar and refrigerate for up to two weeks (use it for dressing pastas, spreading on toast, or topping fresh tomatoes).

CHILLED AND GRILLED OKRA, CORN, AND HEIRLOOM TOMATO SALAD

Yield: 4 to 6 servings
Soundtrack: "Relax Max" by Dinah Washington from *The Swingin' Miss "D"*

After discovering that grilling okra was one way to decrease the slime factor (trust me on this one), I came up with this recipe as a nod to the Southern classic: okra, corn, and tomatoes. I like to serve my version with large, whole romaine lettuce leaves so that folks can stuff them with a few heaping tablespoons of salad and eat it like a taco. I also serve this salad atop **Johnny Blaze Cakes** (page 157).

If you can't grill the corn and okra, you can cook them in the oven. Corn: in its husks (with the silks) at 450°F for about 25 minutes; okra: broiled about 3 inches from the heat, turning with tongs for even cooking, until tender, browned, and lightly crisped, about 14 to 16 minutes.

1 1/2 pounds heirloom tomatoes, diced

1/2 small red onion, diced

1 tablespoon minced basil

1/4 habanero chile, seeded, ribbed, and minced

1 teaspoon freshly squeezed lemon juice

Coarse sea salt

1 tablespoon extra-virgin olive oil

1 pound small-medium okra pods, washed under cold water and dried

18 12-inch wooden skewers, soaked in water for at least 30 minutes

3 large ears sweet corn, silks removed, husks left on, and soaked in cold salted water for 2 hours

Freshly ground black pepper

- Preheat grill.
- In a bowl, combine the tomatoes, onion, basil, chile, lemon juice, 1/2 teaspoon salt, and olive oil and mix well. Cover and refrigerate.
- Thread six or seven okra pods onto two skewers each (to keep the okra in place) and set aside.
- Remove corn from water and place on the grill. Close the cover and grill, turning frequently, until cooked thoroughly, about 20 minutes. Remove from the grill and set aside to cool.

- Transfer the okra to the grill and cook, turning with tongs frequently, until browned and slightly crisped, 6 to 8 minutes.
- Remove from the grill and set aside to cool.
- After the corn and okra have cooled, remove the husks from the corncobs, cut the kernels off the cobs, and add them to a bowl (compost the cobs or save them for broth).

- Cut the okra into $1/2$-inch round slices, discarding the stems, and add them to the bowl with the corn.
- Remove the tomato mixture from the refrigerator. Thoroughly drain the juices and add it to the bowl with the okra and corn.
- Toss the salad well, season with salt and pepper to taste, and serve.

WILD STYLE SALAD (ROCK THE BELLS REMIX)

Yield: 4 to 6 servings

Soundtrack: "Wild" by J Dilla from *Ruff Draft*, "Wild Cowboys" by Sadat X from *Wild Cowboys*, and "Rock the Bells" by LL Cool J from *Radio*

Film: *Wild Style* (1982), directed by Charlie Ahearn. This classic narrative film captures the birth of hip-hop culture in the Bronx, New York.

This remix of my original 2005 Wild Style Salad includes lots of sun-ripened bell peppers, which are crisp and cooling. Wild rice provides a bit of heft to this salad, plus it is rich in protein (twice that of white or brown rice) as well as lots of minerals and B vitamins.

Salad

1 cup wild rice, rinsed and soaked overnight in the refrigerator

1/2 teaspoon fine sea salt

1 green bell pepper, seeded and diced

1 red bell pepper, seeded and diced

1 yellow bell pepper, seeded and diced

1 orange bell pepper, seeded and diced

1/2 cup golden raisins

1/2 cup thinly sliced scallions

1/2 cup cashews, toasted and chopped

Dressing

3 tablespoons apple cider vinegar

1 tablespoon freshly squeezed lemon juice

2 teaspoons Dijon mustard

1 teaspoon agave nectar

1 tablespoon chopped parsley

1/2 teaspoon fine sea salt

1/4 cup extra-virgin olive oil

Freshly ground white pepper

For the salad

- In a medium saucepan over high heat, combine the rice with 3 cups of water and bring to a boil. Add the salt, reduce heat to low, cover, and simmer for 30 minutes.
- Remove from heat, transfer to a strainer or sieve, and rinse under cold water for a few minutes, or until the rice is completely cool.
- In a large bowl, combine the cooked rice, bell pepper, raisins, scallions, and cashews with clean hands.

For the dressing

- In a small bowl, combine the apple cider vinegar, lemon juice, mustard, agave nectar, parsley, and salt. Mix well. Whisk in the olive oil while pouring slowly.
- Pour the dressing over the rice and toss well with clean hands. Cover and refrigerate for 1 hour to allow the flavors to marry.
- Remove rice from the refrigerator 30 minutes before serving.
- Season with white pepper to taste right before serving.

CARAMELIZED GRAPEFRUIT, AVOCADO, AND WATERCRESS SALAD WITH GRAPEFRUIT VINAIGRETTE

Yield: 4 servings
Soundtrack: "Sweet Thing" by Rufus featuring Chaka Khan from *Rufus Featuring Chaka Khan*

One of my major inspirations for this book is food historian Jessica B. Harris's *Welcome Table: African American Heritage Cooking.* Not only does she offer classic African American recipes and family favorite dishes, but she also opens the book with meticulously researched essays on the history and development of African American cuisine. One of the salads that she includes in her book is an "Avocado and Grapefruit Salad." This is the remix. Because of the sweetness from the caramelized grapefruits, I usually enjoy this salad on its own or at the end of a summer meal.

---

4 large grapefruits

1/2 cup organic raw cane sugar

2 teaspoons red wine vinegar

1/2 teaspoon Dijon mustard

1 small clove garlic, minced

1 tablespoon minced fresh mint

Coarse sea salt

7 tablespoons extra-virgin olive oil

Freshly ground white pepper

2 bunches watercress, trimmed of their tough stems

2 large ripe but firm Hass avocados, pitted, peeled, and cut into 1/2-inch cubes

---

- Using a serrated knife, cut a disc off the top and bottom of two of the grapefruits, slicing through the peel and pith to expose the flesh. Set each grapefruit on one cut end and cut downward, following the contours of the fruit, to remove all the skin and the pith, exposing the flesh. Cut the grapefruits crosswise into four even rings and carefully place them on a parchment-lined platter.

- Add the sugar to a medium bowl.

- Warm a large nonstick skillet over high heat.

- While the skillet is heating, dredge the grapefruit slices in the sugar and transfer them back to the platter.

- When the skillet is piping hot, panfry the grapefruit slices for 1½ to 2 minutes each side, until they are golden and caramelized. You may do this in two batches to avoid overcrowding the pan. With a spatula, carefully transfer the grapefruit back to the platter and refrigerate until cold.

- While the grapefruit is cooling, juice the remaining grapefruits and transfer their juice to a small saucepan. Bring to a boil, quickly lower the heat to medium, and simmer to reduce the juice to 3 tablespoons, 8 to 10 minutes. Immediately transfer the juice to an upright blender and set aside to cool.

- Make the vinaigrette by adding the vinegar, mustard, garlic, mint, and ½ teaspoon salt to the blender and slowly pouring in the olive oil with the blender going. Salt and pepper to taste.

- In a large bowl, combine the watercress, the avocado, and enough vinaigrette to lightly coat the salad. Gently toss to coat evenly.

- Divide the salad evenly among four plates. Top each salad with two grapefruit slices and serve immediately.

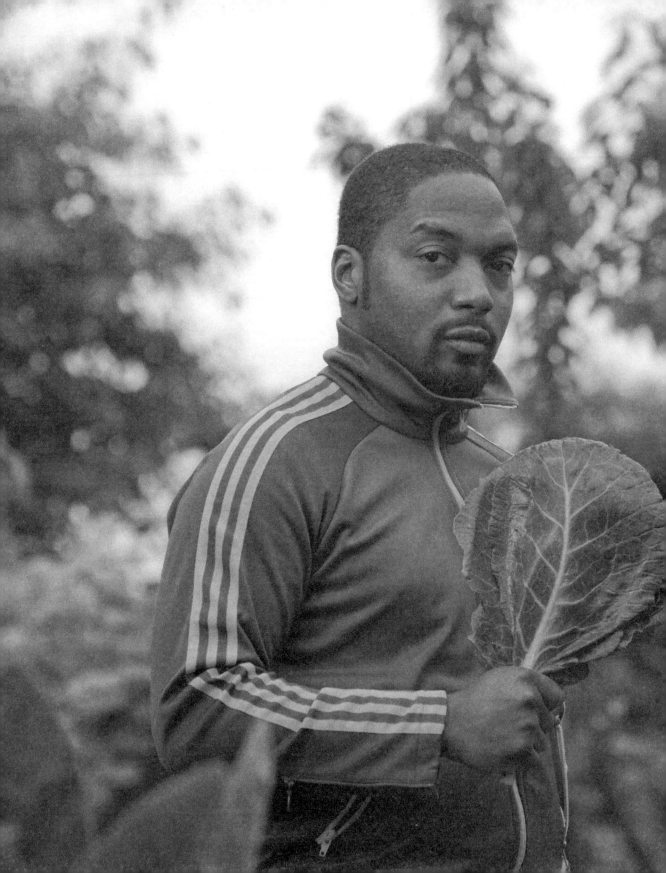

LIQUID LESSONS
SOUPS. STEWS. POT LIKKER.

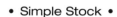

• Simple Stock •

• Garlic Broth •

• Sweet Corn Broth •

• 'Shroom Stock •

• Butternut Squash–Bartlett Pear Soup with
Roasted Butternut Squash Seeds •

• Creamy Yellow Potato Soup with
Rosemary Oil and Crispy Rosemary •

• Charred Plum Tomato and Sweet Corn Soup with
Crispy Okra Strips and a Kick •

• Chilled Heirloom Tomato Soup with
Cucumber Salsa and Toasted Peanuts •

• Cold and Creamy Cucumber-Watermelon Soup with
Pickled Watermelon Rind Salsa •

• Roasted Turnips and Shallots with Turnip Greens Soup •

• Succotash Soup with Garlicky Cornbread Croutons •

• Gumbo Z •

• Roasted Root Vegetable Ital Stew •

• Spicy Mafé Tempeh •

• Tempeh, Shiitake Mushroom, and
Cornmeal Dumpling Stew •

SIMPLE STOCK

Yield: about 1½ quarts
Soundtrack: "Home" by The Modern Jazz Quartet from *Blues at Carnegie Hall*

This stock is all-purpose and can be used whenever a vegetable stock is called for. In addition to the suggested ingredients below, you can add the tough stems and trimmings from leafy greens and other vegetables.

1 tablespoon extra-virgin olive oil

2 large onions, quartered (include skin)

1 large carrot, sliced thinly

4 celery ribs, sliced thinly

8 ounces button mushrooms, sliced thinly (stems included)

1 whole garlic bulb, unpeeled, broken up, and smashed with the back of a knife

2 bay leaves

3 sprigs fresh thyme

½ teaspoon coarse sea salt

⅛ teaspoon cayenne

9 cups water

- In a stockpot over medium-high heat, warm the olive oil. Add the onion, carrot, celery, mushrooms, garlic, bay leaves, thyme, salt, and cayenne and sauté, stirring often, until softened, about 5 minutes. Add the water, bring to a boil, reduce heat to medium-low, and simmer, uncovered, until the vegetables are meltingly tender, about 1 hour.
- Strain the vegetables, pressing down on them to extract all their liquids. Discard (and compost) the cooked vegetables.

STOCKS

Nowadays, I always make my own stocks. It is a good way to use leftover tough stems, trimmings, and the like from vegetables (I freeze these parts in a bag until ready to use), and the qualitative difference is immeasurable. Simply put, homemade stocks are next level. But boxed stocks can work in most of these recipes. All these stocks keep well in the refrigerator for up to two days, and they freeze well.

GARLIC BROTH

Yield: about 1½ quarts
Soundtrack: "Stormy Weather" by
Etta James from *At Last!*

I enjoy combining this sweet, warming
broth with chopped vegetables, herbs, salt,
and pepper to make a simple soup on rainy
days when I don't plan to leave my house.
And I also use it as a quick and easy base
for soups in the fall and winter.

4 whole garlic bulbs, unpeeled, broken
up, and smashed with the back of a
knife
½ teaspoon sea salt
9 cups water

- In a large pot over high heat, combine the
garlic, salt, and water. Bring to a boil, reduce heat to medium-low, and simmer,
uncovered, for about 1 hour.
- Strain the garlic cloves, pressing down on
them to extract all their liquid, and discard
(compost) them.

ROASTING GARLIC

I add roasted garlic to sauces to deepen their flavor, and I spread it on toasted bread
as an appetizer or a snack. To roast it, preheat your oven to 325°F, cut off just enough
of the head of a garlic bulb to expose the garlic cloves, transfer to aluminum foil cut-
side up, and drizzle with extra-virgin olive oil. Wrap the foil tightly, place in a baking
receptacle to catch any drippings, and bake until the garlic is tender, about 1 hour.

SWEET CORN BROTH

Yield: about 1½ quarts
Soundtrack: "I Was a Lover" by TV on the Radio from *Return to Cookie Mountain*

In addition to hydrating by drinking water during the summer, I eat lots of fruits and vegetables with high water content, and I sip broths when it is too hot to have a heavy meal. This is one of my favorites. Simple. To the point. Tasty. I use a lot of fresh corn in the summer, so I started making this broth with all the leftover cobs. After scraping the kernels off of the cobs, store them in a plastic bag in your fridge until you have at least four to make this broth. Minced fresh herbs such as basil, cilantro, and parsley enrich the flavor of this broth when sipping.

4 to 6 cobs from fresh sweet corn, cut or broken in half
9 cups water
Coarse sea salt

- In a medium-size saucepan over high heat, combine the cobs and the water and bring to a boil. Reduce the heat to medium-low and simmer, partially covered, for 45 minutes.
- Strain the broth in a colander and compost the cobs.
- Season with salt to taste and add fresh herbs of your choice if enjoying on its own.

CLEANING MUSHROOMS

I was taught to clean mushrooms by wiping each individual cap with a slightly damp clean kitchen towel. This can be quite tedious, especially when preparing large quantities. So most of the time I quickly wash them in a colander under cold water and wipe off any remaining soil with a clean kitchen towel. As long as your mushrooms do not soak in water, they should be fine.

'SHROOM STOCK

Yield: about 1 1/2 quarts
Soundtrack: "Shroom Music (Champion Bound)" by Quasimoto from *The Further Adventures of Lord Quas*

Whenever I make a dish that requires lots of mushrooms I reserve the stems, freeze them, and pull them out when I'm ready to make this stock. If you do this, estimate how many stems would equal the actual caps suggested in this recipe and substitute. I use this stock as a base for **Tempeh, Shiitake Mushroom, and Cornmeal Dumpling Stew** (page 97) and **Mixed Mushroom Gravy** (page 181), which goes over **Smothered Seitan Medallions in Mixed-Mushroom Gravy** (page 153).

1 tablespoon extra-virgin olive oil

1 large onion, diced (include skin)

1 large carrot, sliced thinly

4 celery ribs, sliced thinly

1 pound button mushrooms (stems included), sliced thinly

1 pound portobello mushrooms (stems included), sliced thinly

2 ounces dried shiitake mushrooms

1/2 garlic bulb, unpeeled, broken up, and crushed

2 bay leaves

3 sprigs fresh thyme

1/8 teaspoon cayenne

1/2 teaspoon coarse sea salt

9 cups water

- In a stockpot over medium-high heat, warm the olive oil. Add the onion, carrot, celery, mushrooms, garlic, bay leaves, thyme, cayenne, and salt and sauté, stirring often, until softened, about 5 minutes. Add the water, bring to a boil, reduce heat to medium-low, and simmer, uncovered for about 1 hour, until the vegetables are meltingly tender.

- Strain the vegetables, pressing down on them to extract all their juices. Compost the cooked vegetables.

BUTTERNUT SQUASH–BARTLETT PEAR SOUP WITH ROASTED BUTTERNUT SQUASH SEEDS

Yield: 4 to 6 servings
Soundtrack: "Summer Sun" by Koop (Markus Enochson Remix) from *Waltz for Koop—Alternative Takes*

In the summer of 2006 I was invited to do a cooking demonstration at the downtown farmers' market in Memphis. They asked me to submit a recipe in advance, but I told them I wouldn't know what I would cook until that morning when I visited the market and saw what was available. A farmer from Arkansas was selling beautiful Bartlett pears, and I decided to use them to make this soup. That day, I used heavy cream, but coconut milk gives it an equally creamy, satisfying flavor.

———

PUREEING SOUPS

The easiest way to make a creamy soup is to puree it with an immersion blender. But I prefer using a traditional upright blender since I have always done it that way. If you do use an upright blender, be sure not to fill it more than halfway and cover the top with a clean kitchen towel to protect yourself from any splattering.

3 tablespoons extra-virgin olive oil

2 medium leeks (white and tender green parts), chopped finely

1 small butternut squash (about 2 pounds), peeled, seeded, and cut into 1-inch pieces (seeds reserved)

3 Bartlett pears (about 1½ pounds), peeled and chopped into roughly 1-inch pieces

5 cups **Simple Stock** (page 76)

Coarse sea salt

1 14-ounce can coconut milk

2 sprigs thyme, minced

Freshly ground white pepper

Roasted butternut squash seeds (page 43), for garnish

- In a medium-size saucepan over medium-low heat, warm the olive oil. Add the leeks and cook, stirring often, until they are soft, 8 to 10 minutes.

- Add the squash and pears and cook for 5 minutes. Add the Simple Stock and bring to a boil. Lower the heat, add ½ teaspoon salt, and simmer, stirring often, until the squash is fork tender, about 20 minutes.

- Stir in the coconut milk, then puree the soup in batches in an upright blender or with an immersion blender. Add the soup back to the saucepan, add the thyme, and warm over medium-low heat for a few minutes. Season with white pepper and salt to taste. Served garnished with roasted butternut squash seeds.

CREAMY YELLOW POTATO SOUP WITH ROSEMARY OIL AND CRISPY ROSEMARY

Yield: 4 to 6 servings

Soundtrack: "Greens at the Chicken Shack" by Roy Hargrove Quintet from *With the Tenors of Our Time*

Eat this easy-to-make soup with crusty bread on winter nights. The fragrant, crispy rosemary gives it a pretty presentation.

- -

3 tablespoons extra-virgin olive oil

3 2-inch sprigs of rosemary

2 large yellow onions

1 teaspoon cumin

Coarse sea salt

3 cloves garlic, minced

6 cups **Simple Stock** (page 76) or **Garlic Broth** (page 77)

2 pounds Yukon Gold potatoes, peeled and diced

White pepper

- -

- In a medium-size saucepan over high heat, warm the olive oil until hot but not smoking, about 1 minute. Turn off the heat and immediately remove the rosemary from the sprigs into the hot oil and cook until crispy, shaking the pan to ensure that all the rosemary is covered in oil. Strain the oil into a small bowl, set the crispy rosemary aside, and return the oil back to the saucepan.

- Add the onions, cumin, and 1/4 teaspoon of salt to the saucepan, turn on the heat to medium-high, and sauté until soft, about 5 minutes. Add the garlic and sauté until fragrant, about 1 1/2 minutes.

- Add the Simple Stock, potatoes, and 1/2 teaspoon of salt and bring to a boil over high heat. Reduce the heat to medium, and simmer, covered, until the potatoes are tender, about 25 minutes.

- Transfer the soup, in batches, to an upright blender and purée until creamy.

- Strain through a medium-mesh sieve and return back to the saucepan.

- Season with salt and pepper to taste and add additional stock to thin, if necessary. Serve hot, garnishing each bowl with crispy rosemary.

CHARRED PLUM TOMATO AND SWEET CORN SOUP WITH CRISPY OKRA STRIPS AND A KICK

Yield: 4 to 6 servings

Soundtrack: "Sun Is Shining" by Bob Marley and The Wailers from *The Complete Upsetter Collection*

With an eye on one of my favorite summer dishes—roasted plum tomatoes and garlic—I decided to flip the classic okra, corn, and tomatoes combination once more, but this time into a soup. Some dishes require that you only use the freshest seasonal ingredients. This is one of them.

- -

8 large plum tomatoes, halved

10 large cloves garlic (unpeeled)

4 tablespoons extra-virgin olive oil plus more for drizzling the tomatoes

2 large ears yellow corn, shucked, kernels scraped, cobs cut in half and reserved (cobs can be used to make broth for this dish)

Coarse sea salt

1 large yellow onion, diced

1/2 teaspoon crushed red pepper flakes

6 cups **Sweet Corn Broth** (page 78)

Freshly ground white pepper

Crispy Okra Strips with Lime-Thyme Vinaigrette (page 46)

- -

- Preheat the oven to 450°F.
- Place the tomatoes, cut side up, on a parchment-lined baking sheet and place the garlic cloves in between them. Drizzle the tomatoes with olive oil. Bake for about 45 minutes, until the tomatoes have softened and are starting to char around the edges. Remove from the oven and set aside to cool.
- In a small sauté pan over medium heat, combine the corn kernels, 1/4 teaspoon of sea salt, and 1 tablespoon of olive oil and sauté, stirring occasionally, until the corn is tender, about 5 minutes. Remove from heat and set aside.
- In a medium-size saucepan over medium heat, combine the onions, the red pepper flakes, 1/4 teaspoon of sea salt, and 1 tablespoon of olive oil and sauté until translucent, about 5 minutes.
- Peel the garlic cloves and add them along with the tomatoes (and their juices), the remaining olive oil, 1 teaspoon of sea salt, and the broth to the saucepan with the onion mixture. Cook for 2 minutes, stirring constantly to incorporate.
- Puree the soup in batches in an upright blender or with an immersion blender. Strain through a medium mesh strainer and return back to the saucepan. Stir in the corn kernels, puree again in batches in an upright blender or with an immersion blender, and return back to the saucepan (don't strain the second time). Season with white pepper and salt to taste.
- Allow the soup to cool to room temperature, ladle into bowls, and garnish with a few cakes of crispy okra strips.

CHILLED HEIRLOOM TOMATO SOUP WITH CUCUMBER SALSA AND TOASTED PEANUTS

Yield: 4 to 6 servings
Soundtrack: "Sea Lion Woman" by Feist from *The Reminder*

With the increasing chorus of voices calling for more biodiversity in our food system, heirloom tomatoes have become popular and more readily available over the past decade. While the bizarre shapes and unusual colors of heirloom tomatoes might throw off newcomers, their varied tastes and textures keep folks coming back for more. The cool thing about this soup is that there are endless flavor possibilities depending on what variety of tomato you use. Remix this soup by using different varieties every time you make it and enjoy it chilled or at room temperature.

And speaking of (re)mixes, I have to big-up chefs Alice Waters and Peter Berley for inspiring this recipe. When I was brainstorming ideas for summer soups, I ran across a recipe for Chilled Tomato Soup with Shallots, Cucumbers, and Corn in Peter's book *Fresh Food Fast*. In the headnote, he tells us that Alice's Gazpacho inspired his soup. I hope this soup inspires someone to remix it.

Cucumber Salsa

1 large cucumber, peeled, seeded,
    and diced

1/2 cup diced red onion

1 clove garlic, minced

2 teaspoons minced fresh basil

2 tablespoons freshly squeezed
    lemon juice (from 1 lemon)

1/4 teaspoon coarse sea salt

1/2 teaspoon paprika

2 teaspoons extra-virgin olive oil

Soup

3 1/2 pounds heirloom tomatoes
    (preferably a single variety), cut into
    1-inch slices

2 teaspoons coarse sea salt

1/2 cup toasted peanuts, for garnish
    (page 41)

For the salsa

- In a medium-size bowl, combine all the ingredients and stir well. Set aside.

For the soup

- In a large bowl, toss the tomatoes with 2 teaspoons of salt to enhance their flavor and help release their juices. Cover and set aside for 30 minutes.

- Add the tomatoes to an upright blender and puree until creamy. Strain the liquid into a large bowl, discarding the solids.

- To serve, ladle the soup into bowls and, with a slotted spoon, transfer a heaping tablespoon of cucumber salsa to each bowl. Finish off with a heaping tablespoon of toasted peanuts for garnish.

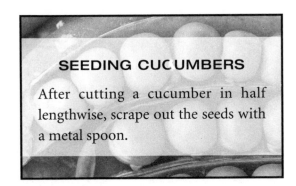

SEEDING CUCUMBERS

After cutting a cucumber in half lengthwise, scrape out the seeds with a metal spoon.

COLD AND CREAMY CUCUMBER-WATERMELON SOUP WITH PICKLED WATERMELON RIND SALSA

Yield: 4 to 6 servings

Soundtrack: "Ease Your Mind" by Goapele featuring Pep Love from *Even Closer*

The main ingredients in this soup—cucumber and watermelon—contain the highest percentage of water of all the fruits and vegetables. This makes it the perfect cooling and hydrating meal to enjoy on scorching hot summer days. Along with the cucumber, the yellow watermelon gives this soup a beautiful lime color. If yellow watermelon is not available, red will do.

Salsa

- 1 cup **Citrus and Spice Pickled Watermelon Rind** (page 20), cut into 1/2-inch dice
- 1/4 cup diced red onion
- 1 tablespoon fresh cilantro
- 1/2 teaspoon freshly squeezed lemon juice

Soup

- 2 cups cubed yellow watermelon
- 5 cups peeled, seeded, and chopped cucumbers (about 5 medium cucumbers)
- 1/4 to 1/2 small habanero chile, seeded and minced
- 1 tablespoon red wine vinegar
- 1 tablespoon extra-virgin olive oil
- 3/4 teaspoon coarse sea salt
- Freshly ground white pepper

For the salsa

- Combine the ingredients in a small bowl, toss well, cover, and refrigerate.

For the soup

- Add the watermelon cubes to an upright blender and puree until smooth. Strain through a medium-mesh strainer to remove seeds and return the juice back to the blender. Add the cucumber and puree until smooth. Add the chile, vinegar, olive oil, and 3/4 teaspoon of salt and puree until smooth. Season with white pepper to taste.
- Pour into chilled bowls, add a dollop or two of salsa, and serve.

ROASTED TURNIPS AND SHALLOTS WITH TURNIP GREENS SOUP

Yield: 4 to 6 servings
Soundtrack: "Turnip's Big Move" by The Greyboy Allstars from *A Town Called Earth*
Art: "Grounded" by Leslie Hewitt

I first made this dish on one of those Saturdays where it was clear that winter was over and spring had finally arrived to stay. After getting all the ingredients from the farmers' market near my house, I came home, cooked it, and ate while sitting on the floor with all the windows in my house wide open. This is a great spring soup since turnips are good for general detoxification. They are also full of nutrients, including vitamins B and C, potassium, phosphorus, calcium, and other trace nutrients.

2 bunches of young turnips with greens

3 medium shallots, peeled and cut into 1/2-inch pieces

2 teaspoons extra-virgin olive oil

Fine sea salt

3 cloves garlic, minced

1 2-inch sprig rosemary

6 cups **Simple Stock** (page 76)

White pepper

- Preheat the oven to 400°F.
- Trim the roots from the turnips and cut into 1/2-inch pieces. Set the greens aside. In a medium-size bowl, toss the turnip pieces and shallots with 1 teaspoon of the olive oil and 1/4 teaspoon of salt. Spread them in a parchment-lined baking dish and roast for 1 hour, stirring every 15 minutes for even browning.
- While the turnips are roasting, trim and discard the tough stems from the greens. Chop them into bite-size pieces, rinse well, and drain. Combine 1 teaspoon of olive oil and the garlic in a large saucepan over medium heat. Sauté for 1 1/2 minutes, until fragrant, then add the greens and 1/4 teaspoon salt. Sauté the greens until tender, stirring occasionally, about 5 minutes. Add the Simple Stock to the saucepan and set aside.
- When the turnips and shallots are done roasting, transfer them to the saucepan. Add the rosemary. Bring to a boil, then lower to a simmer and cook for 5 minutes. Add white pepper and salt to taste. Serve hot.

SUCCOTASH SOUP WITH GARLICKY CORNBREAD CROUTONS

Yield: 4 to 6 servings
Soundtrack: "Succotash" by Herbie Hancock from *Inventions & Dimensions*

Succotash, a Native American dish consisting primarily of lima beans and corn, has been reinterpreted by Southern African Americans with a number of bean-vegetable-and-sometimes-meat combinations. Here I remix the simplest version of this dish by making a tasty pureed soup. While you can get away with using frozen lima beans for this dish, using fresh corn-off-the-cob is essential. So enjoy it during the summer months when corn is at its freshest.

2 cups fresh baby lima beans, rinsed (use frozen if fresh are unavailable)
10 cups cold water
Coarse sea salt
4 large ears yellow corn, shucked, kernels scraped, cobs reserved
1/4 cup plus 1/2 teaspoon extra-virgin olive oil
1 large onion, diced
1/4 cup finely chopped flat-leaf parsley
White pepper
Garlicky Cornbread Croutons (page 156)

- In a medium-size saucepan, combine the beans with the water. Bring to a boil. Reduce the heat to medium, partially cover, and simmer for about 10 minutes, or until the beans are slightly tender. Add 1 teaspoon salt and simmer for 5 more minutes. Drain the cooking liquid into a bowl, set the beans aside, and add the liquid back to the saucepan.

- To make a broth, cut the corncobs into thirds, add them to the bean liquid, and bring to a boil. Reduce the heat to medium-low, partially cover, and simmer for 30 minutes. Remove from heat. With a slotted spoon, remove the corncobs from the liquid to a compost pail.

- While the broth is simmering: in a medium-size sauté pan over medium-low heat, combine the olive oil, 1/4 teaspoon salt, and the onions and sweat for 15 minutes, until the onions are softened. Set aside 1/3 cup of corn kernels and add the rest to the onions. Cook for about 5 minutes, stirring occasionally, until the corn is tender.

- Transfer the corn-onion mixture to the broth. Add the cooked beans. Over high heat, bring to a boil, immediately reduce heat to medium-low, and simmer for 5 more minutes, until the corn is done.

- Remove from heat, stir in 2 tablespoons of the parsley, and puree in small batches in an upright blender. Strain through a medium-mesh strainer to remove tough corn skins. Season with salt and pepper to taste and set aside.

- Preheat broiler. In a small bowl, toss the reserved corn kernels with 1/2 teaspoon of olive oil. Transfer kernels to a 9-inch pie pan or comparable receptacle. Place the corn about 3 inches from the heat and broil until browned, about 3 to 5 minutes, stirring a few times with a spoon.

- If necessary, warm up the soup, then ladle it into bowls, sprinkle roasted corn kernels and Garlicky Cornbread Croutons on top, and garnish with the remaining parsley.

GUMBO Z

Yield: 4 to 6 servings
Soundtrack: "Back Water Blues" by Irma Thomas from *Our New Orleans*

Gumbo des Herbes a.k.a. Gumbo Z'Herbs a.k.a. Gumbo Zav was traditionally eaten as a nonmeat dish during the Roman Catholic season of Lent. In addition to roux, which is used in many traditional gumbos as a thickener, Gumbo Zav included a combination of several greens (sometimes up to nine), along with other vegetables. As time passed, seafood and meats were also included in the dish to season it and add animal protein. But I'm taking it back to the old school with this one.

While I heard a lot about Gumbo Zav when I lived in New Orleans, I never tried it until I visited the city years after I moved away. Since I didn't eat pork, I just picked out the pieces of sausage that were floating around in the stew and dived in. That all-green gumbo was scrumptious and deeply satisfying. I felt so nourished after eating those nutrient-dense greens and drinking that belly-warming pot likker, I decided to create my own version—Gumbo Z.

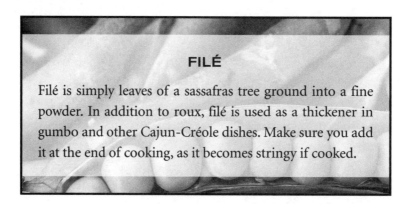

FILÉ

Filé is simply leaves of a sassafras tree ground into a fine powder. In addition to roux, filé is used as a thickener in gumbo and other Cajun-Créole dishes. Make sure you add it at the end of cooking, as it becomes stringy if cooked.

Coarse sea salt

1 large bunch collard greens
(about 1 pound), trimmed and
chopped into bite-size pieces

1 large bunch mustard greens
(about 1 pound), trimmed and
chopped into bite-size pieces

1 large bunch kale (about 1/2 pound),
trimmed and chopped into bite-size
pieces

1 large bunch spinach (about 11/2
pounds), trimmed and chopped into
bite-size pieces

1/2 cup extra-virgin olive oil

7 cloves garlic, minced

1/2 cup whole wheat pastry flour

2 large yellow onions, cut into
1/4 inch dice

2 large red bell peppers, cut into
1/4 inch dice

2 celery ribs, halved lengthwise and
chopped

1/4 teaspoon cayenne

6 cups **Simple Stock** (page 76)

1 tablespoon minced fresh thyme

1 teaspoon filé

1 tablespoon **Hot Apple Cider Vinegar**
(page 165)

2 large scallions, sliced thinly, for garnish

- In a large pot over high heat, bring 4 quarts of water to a boil. Add 1 tablespoon of salt.

- Add all the leafy greens to the water, bring back to a boil, and cook uncovered, for 3 to 4 minutes, until the sulfur has escaped. Drain in a colander and cool.

- Transfer the greens to a cutting board and chop well.

- Combine 1/4 cup of the olive oil with the garlic in a large sauté pan over medium heat and sauté until fragrant and starting to turn golden, about 2 minutes. Add the greens mixture, raise the heat to high, sprinkle with 1 teaspoon of salt, and sauté, stirring occasionally, for 2 to 3 minutes, until well coated with oil. Set aside.

- In a large pot over the lowest heat possible, combine the flour and the remaining olive oil and cook, stirring often with a wooden spoon, until caramel colored, about 25 minutes. Add the onion, bell peppers, celery, cayenne, and 1/2 teaspoon of salt. Raise the heat to medium and sauté, stirring occasionally and scraping the bottom of the pot, until the vegetables soften, about 15 minutes. Slowly stir in the stock. Add the reserved greens, bring to a boil, and reduce the heat to low. Cover and simmer until meltingly tender, about 45 minutes.

- Stir in the thyme and simmer for an additional 2 minutes. Remove from heat, stir in the filé and the Hot Apple Cider Vinegar, and set aside to cool for 10 minutes.

- Serve garnished with scallions over long-grain brown rice.

GUMBO

Granny was God in the kitchen
Her ladle
sunk deep in swamp green
Ground brown
Grey soup
vanished
and came up full
a mound of sea creatures
A crab leg reached over the lip
Out of the primordial roux
Granny turned and filled my bowl
Gumbo swirled around its parts
And left a spiraling galaxy of spice
In my warm palms
Its scent
swaddled in my own breath
soaked my tongue in savory
And when Granny looked down
at what she made
She knew it was good

—Michael Otieno Molina

ROASTED ROOT VEGETABLE ITAL STEW

Yield: 6 to 8 servings

Soundtrack: "Don't Cry" by Dezarie from *FYA*

Film: *Country Man* (1982), directed by Dickie Jobson. This narrative film follows a Jamaican Rastafarian fisherman with mystical powers and chronicles his adventures.

Derived from the word "vital," "Ital" is employed throughout Rastafari jargon as a way to emphasize the oneness and unity of life. Ital food promotes a healthy mind, body, spirit, and environment. It is as fresh as possible; free from additives, preservatives, and other chemicals; and in most cases dairy free. Many Ital dishes are Caribbean-inspired, but any recipe can be Ital if it is prepared in accordance with Rasta principles. This stew is perfect on cool fall and winter evenings.

---

1 cup dried kidney beans

5 2-inch slices of ginger

1 3-inch piece kombu

Coarse sea salt

2 cups peeled and diced winter squash (such as kabocha, acorn, or butternut)

1/2 cup peeled and diced parsnips

1 cup peeled and diced sweet potato

1 cup peeled and diced Yukon Gold potatoes

5 tablespoons extra-virgin olive oil

1 large onion, diced

1 teaspoon dried thyme

1 teaspoon ground allspice

1/8 teaspoon cayenne

1 habanero chile, seeded and minced

10 cloves roasted garlic (page 77)

2 cups **Simple Stock** (page 76)

1 cup long beans, sliced into 2-inch diagonals

2 cups quartered Brussels sprouts

1 14-ounce can coconut milk

1 teaspoon agave nectar

1 tablespoon freshly squeezed lime juice

1/2 cup minced cilantro

Freshly ground white pepper

- Preheat the oven to 450°F.
- Combine the kidney beans, ginger, and kombu with enough water to cover them by two inches in a medium-size saucepan over medium heat and bring to a boil. Skim off any foam, reduce the heat to medium-low, and simmer, partially covered, until the beans are starting to turn tender, about 40 minutes, adding more water as needed to keep the beans covered. Add 1 teaspoon salt and cook for an additional 10 minutes. Drain the beans, reserving their cooking liquid.
- Meanwhile, in a large bowl, toss the squash, parsnips, sweet potatoes, and potatoes with 3 tablespoons of olive oil and 1/2 teaspoon salt.
- Spread the vegetables on a parchment-lined baking sheet and roast for about 50 minutes, stirring every 15 minutes for even browning, until the vegetables are tender and caramelized.
- While the beans are cooking and the vegetables are roasting, combine 2 tablespoons of olive oil with the onions, thyme, allspice, cayenne, and 1/2 teaspoon salt in a large saucepan and cook for 10 minutes, stirring often, until vegetables are soft. Add the chile and garlic and cook for an additional 2 minutes.
- Add the reserved beans, 2 cups of the reserved bean liquid, the roasted vegetables, and the Simple Stock to the saucepan and bring to a simmer over medium-low heat. Simmer, partially covered, for 35 minutes, stirring occasionally. Add the long beans and Brussels sprouts and simmer for an additional 10 minutes, until soft. Stir in the coconut milk, agave nectar, lime juice, and cilantro and simmer until heated through, about 3 more minutes.
- Season with salt and pepper to taste. Serve with **Brown Coconut Rice** (page 126)

SPICY MAFÉ TEMPEH

Yield: 4 to 6 servings
Soundtrack: "Ma Hine Cocore (3rd Bass Remix by Yossi Fine)" by Vieux Farka Touré from *Remixed: UFOs over Bamako*
Art: "MAOBOLEZO YA MAWAZO NA NYSY" by Githinji Wa Mbire

Originally from the border of Mali, Mafé is a traditional stew of the Wolof people of Senegal, West Africa. It is often made with lamb, but it can also be made with beef, chicken, or fish. In most of the Senegalese restaurants that I have visited, the vegetarian version uses tofu. Here, I use tempeh. Its nutty flavor goes well with the peanut base of this dish. In case you don't know, peanuts are an important staple to the Wolof people, as a great number of them make their living as peanut farmers.

2 cups raw shelled peanuts

2 jalapeños

6 cups **Simple Stock** (page 76)

Coarse sea salt

1/2 pound (1 8-ounce package) tempeh, cut into 1/2-inch cubes

1 tablespoon peanut oil

1 medium yellow onion, diced

4 large carrots, sliced thinly on the diagonal

1/2 cup unsalted creamy peanut butter (preferably fresh)

1/3 cup tomato paste

1 cup canned diced tomatoes with their juices

3 cups sliced red cabbage

2 teaspoons freshly squeezed lemon juice

Freshly ground white pepper

1/2 cup **Spicy Goobers** (page 42) for garnish

1/2 cup chopped parsley

- Preheat the oven to 350°F.
- To make a marinade, in an upright blender combine the peanuts, 1 jalapeño, 3 cups of the Simple Stock, and 1 teaspoon salt. Blend well, about 1 minute. In a large bowl, combine the mixture with 2 cups of water and stir well with a spoon.
- Pour half of the marinade into a baking dish that can hold the tempeh cubes in a single snug layer. Place the tempeh on top and pour on the remaining marinade.
- Tightly cover the dish with foil and bake for 1 hour.
- While the tempeh is cooking, warm the peanut oil in a 4-quart saucepan over medium heat. Add the onions and a 1/4 teaspoon of salt, reduce the heat to low, and cook for 10 minutes, stirring occasionally. Add the carrots and cook for about 5 minutes. Remove from heat and set aside.

- In an upright blender, combine the peanut butter, the tomato paste, the remaining jalapeño (remove seeds and spines for less heat), and 1 1/2 cups stock. Blend well and add to the saucepan with the vegetables. Add the tomatoes and the remaining stock to the saucepan.
- When it is done cooking, immediately remove the tempeh from the oven, drain the pieces into a colander shaking the pan to remove the marinade, and transfer the pieces to the saucepan.
- Raise the heat and bring to a boil. Reduce the heat to low and simmer gently, uncovered, until the stew has thickened, 45 minutes to 1 hour.
- Add the cabbage and lemon juice and cook just until the cabbage is soft, about 3 minutes.
- Season with salt and pepper to taste and serve garnished with Spicy Goobers and parsley along with brown rice.

TEMPEH, SHIITAKE MUSHROOM, AND CORNMEAL DUMPLING STEW

Yield: 6 to 8 servings

Soundtrack: "Chicken an' Dumplins" by Art Blakey & The Jazz Messengers from *At the Jazz Corner of the World*

I created this dish in hopes of conjuring up memories of my mom's homemade chicken and dumplings. Here's to simpler days.

Dumplings

5 cups water

1/2 cup whole wheat pastry flour

1/2 cup cornmeal

2 teaspoons ground flaxseed

1 1/2 teaspoons baking powder

1/2 teaspoon fine sea salt

1 tablespoon extra-virgin olive oil

3 tablespoons cold, unflavored rice milk

Stew

1 cup extra-virgin olive oil

1 pound (2 8-ounce packages) tempeh, sliced into 1/2-inch fingers, then sliced in half widthwise

2 medium leeks (white and tender green parts), chopped finely

2 tablespoons finely chopped shallot

1/2 teaspoon red pepper flakes

Coarse sea salt

8 1/2 ounces shiitake mushrooms, sliced thinly

2 large celery ribs with leaves, sliced thinly

2 medium carrots, sliced thinly on the diagonal

2 tablespoons whole wheat pastry flour

6 cups **'Shroom Stock** (page 79)

1/2 cup silken tofu

1 tablespoon minced thyme

1 tablespoon freshly squeezed lemon juice

Freshly ground white pepper

For the dumplings

- In a medium-size saucepan, bring the water to a boil.

- In the meantime, sift together the flour, cornmeal, ground flaxseed, baking powder, and salt in a medium-size bowl. Make a well in the center of the dry mixture, add the olive oil and rice milk, and stir quickly just until the dough comes away from the sides of the bowl.

- Reduce heat under saucepan to lowest simmer. Gently drop tablespoons of the batter into the simmering water with a tiny ice cream scoop or a tablespoon, waiting about 15 seconds in between each drop. Cover and simmer for 10 minutes.

- When they are done, *gently* remove each dumpling with a slotted spoon to a plate and set aside. Discard the water in the saucepan.

For the stew

- While the dumplings are simmering, warm the olive oil in a medium-size skillet over medium-high heat. Add half of the tempeh fingers and cook for 3 to 5 minutes, until golden brown. Turn the fingers over, and cook for 3 to 5 minutes more, until lightly browned on the other side. With a slotted spatula, transfer the tempeh to a large plate lined with paper towels.

- Pour off most of the olive oil from the skillet (reserve in a small bowl), leaving a thin film on the bottom. Add the leeks, shallot, red pepper flakes, and 1 teaspoon salt to the skillet and slowly sauté over medium-low heat. Cook until soft, stirring often to prevent burning, about 5 minutes. Add the mushrooms, celery, and carrots and cook for 5 more minutes. Push all the vegetables to the side of the pan, leaving space in the middle. Add 1 tablespoon of the reserved olive oil and 2 tablespoons of whole wheat pastry flour to the center of the pan. Stir with a spoon to mix well. Add 1 cup of the stock, mix everything in the pan well to combine, and cook at a simmer until starting to thicken, about 5 minutes.

- Transfer all of the ingredients in the skillet to the saucepan that was used for the dumplings. Add the remaining 'Shroom Stock and the tempeh fingers and bring to a simmer. Reduce the heat to low, cover, and simmer for 20 minutes. With a ladle, remove 1 cup of the broth from the saucepan and transfer to an upright blender. Add the tofu and blend until creamy. Pour this mixture into the saucepan, and simmer for 10 more minutes.

- Stir in the thyme and lemon juice. Simmer for 1 minute, then season with salt and white pepper to taste.

- Serve each bowl of stew with a few dumplings on top.

CLEANING LEEKS

First cut off the green tops, leaving only the light green and white bottom. Cut off the roots. Slice the leek in half lengthwise, then slice horizontally. Fill a large bowl with cold water, add the leek slices, and swish around vigorously, rubbing any residue off the pieces. Rinse the bowl of any residue and repeat if necessary.

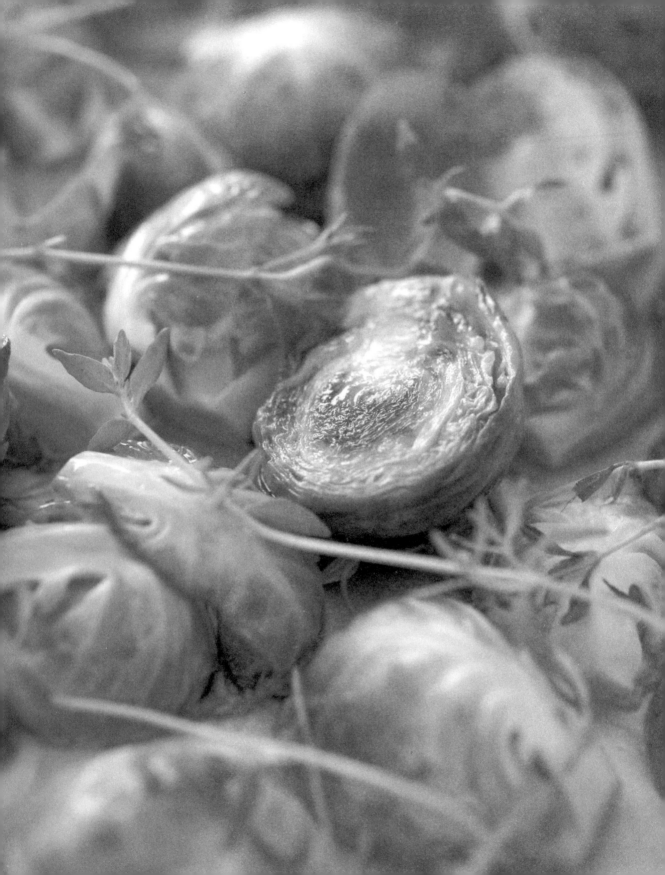

SO FRESH AND SO GREEN GREEN
VERITABLE VEGETABLES

• Simple Seared Green Beans •

• Grilled Asparagus with Rosemary Sea Salt •

• Grilled Corn on the Cob with Spicy Garlic-Miso Dressing •

• Mixed-Herb-Marinated Grilled Summer
Squash and Bell Peppers •

• Green Pea and Leek Puree •

• Sautéed Jalapeño Corn •

• Sweet Coconut-Ginger Creamed Corn •

• Crisp Green Beans with Roasted Shallots and Walnuts •

• Fried Green Tomatoes with Creamy Celeriac Sauce •

• Jamaican Veggie Patties •

• Roasted Root Vegetables with Roasted Garlic–Lime Dipping Sauce •

• Roasted Sweet Potato Puree with Coconut Milk •

• Cumin-Cayenne Mashed Potatoes with Caramelized Onions •

• Little Potato and Sweet Potato Pancakes •

• Candied Sweet Potato Discs and Apple Slices •

• Collard Confetti •

• Spicy Smothered Green Cabbage •

• Wilted Swiss Chard and Spinach with Lemon-Tahini Dressing •

• Garlic Broth–Braised Brussels Sprouts •

• Roasted Potato and Mixed Greens Gratin •

Spring and Summer

SIMPLE SEARED GREEN BEANS

Yield: 4 to 6 servings
Soundtrack: "Lay It Down" by Al Green featuring Anthony Hamilton from
Lay It Down

Most of the time, the best way to enjoy vegetables at the height of freshness is to prepare them as simply as possible so that the main ingredient can shine. Here I blanch green beans, sear them in **Garlic Olive Oil** (page 166), and dust them with sea salt.

½ teaspoon coarse sea salt

1½ pounds fresh green beans, snapped at each end

1 tablespoon **Garlic Olive Oil** (page 166)

- Bring 4 quarts of water to a boil in a large pot over high heat and add 1 tablespoon of salt. Add the green beans and cook 2 to 3 minutes, until tender but al dente. Drain the green beans into a colander and shock in a bowl filled with ice water. Drain again and pat dry.

- In a large skillet or a wok over high heat, heat the Garlic Olive Oil until hot, add the green beans and ½ teaspoon of sea salt, and cook, tossing constantly, until coated with olive oil and cooked through, about 3 minutes.

- Serve immediately.

GRILLED ASPARAGUS WITH ROSEMARY SEA SALT

Yield: 4 servings
Soundtrack: "Escape That" by 4hero from *Two Pages*

Grilling is one of my favorite ways to prepare asparagus—the harbinger of spring—and celebrate the end of winter. If you don't want to break out your grill before summer hits, you can also roast it in the oven at 400°F until it starts to crisp, 8 to 10 minutes. I also serve this dish topped with a few dollops of **Creamy Celeriac Sauce** (page 170).

1 tablespoon coarse sea salt

1 pound asparagus, rinsed and trimmed

1 tablespoon extra-virgin olive oil

Herbed Sea Salt (rosemary) (page 162)

Freshly ground white pepper

1 large lemon, cut in half

- Light the grill.
- In a large pot over high heat, bring 4 quarts of water to a boil. Add 1 tablespoon of salt, boil for 1 minute, add the asparagus, and immediately turn off the heat. Let sit for 1 minute, then drain.
- Transfer the asparagus to a large plate and toss in the olive oil to coat lightly.
- Transfer the asparagus to the grill and cook, turning the spears with tongs for even cooking, until tender and slightly charred, 3 to 4 minutes.
- Transfer the asparagus back to the plate, dust with the rosemary salt and white pepper, and squeeze with lemon juice.

GRILLED CORN ON THE COB WITH SPICY GARLIC-MISO DRESSING

Yield: 4 servings
Soundtrack: "Summer Rain" by Smokey & Miho from *The Two EPs*

This garlic-miso dressing provides enough creaminess and flavor to make this corn on the cob equally satisfying as the drowned-in-butter variety. When I serve this version at family cookouts, most of my family members prefer it to buttered corn. You can also roast these in the oven at 450°F for 10 to 15 minutes.

Coarse sea salt

4 large ears corn (leave on silks and husks)

2 tablespoons freshly squeezed lemon juice

2 tablespoons apple cider vinegar

1/4 cup mellow white miso

2 tablespoons extra-virgin olive oil

1 teaspoon agave nectar

1 jalapeño (seeds included), topped and trimmed

3 cloves garlic, minced

1/8 teaspoon cayenne

Freshly ground white pepper

1/4 teaspoon paprika

- Fill a large container in which the corn can be submerged under water. Add 2 tablespoons of salt and stir until dissolved. Add the corn, submerge, and soak for at least 2 hours.
- Light the grill.
- When the grill is hot, transfer the corncobs to a rack and cook, turning occasionally with tongs, for about 25 minutes.
- Meanwhile, in an upright blender, combine the lemon juice, vinegar, miso, olive oil, agave nectar, jalapeño, garlic, cayenne, and 1/4 teaspoon salt and blend until creamy. Transfer to a large bowl, and set aside.
- When the corn is done, remove the husks, transfer the cobs to the bowl with the dressing, and toss until well coated.
- Season with salt and white pepper to taste and dust with paprika before serving.

MIXED-HERB-MARINATED GRILLED SUMMER SQUASH AND BELL PEPPERS

Yield: 4 to 6 servings
Soundtrack: "Sarsaparilla" by MF DOOM from *Metal Fingers Presents . . . Special Herbs Vols. 7&8*

Grilling vegetables is one of the easiest ways to feed a lot of folks at summer cookouts. You can also cook these under a broiler, placing them about 6 inches from the heat for 6 to 8 minutes, until charred. I sometimes add button mushrooms, squares of tofu, and onions chopped into big chunks to the marinade; then I thread the vegetables onto skewers for kabobs. You can drain the marinade of any solids and freeze it for later use.

Mixed-Herb Marinade (page 169), doubled

1½ pounds mixed summer squash, cut into ½-inch lengthwise slices

1 large red bell pepper

1 large yellow bell pepper

1 large orange bell pepper

- In a large bowl, combine the marinade with the vegetables and refrigerate for at least 3 hours or overnight, tossing occasionally.
- Light your grill.
- Grill the squash and peppers over high heat, turning occasionally, until charred.
- Transfer the squash to a serving platter.
- Peel the peppers of their charred skins and discard the skin, seeds, and stem. Cut the peppers in half lengthwise. Transfer them to the serving platter with the squash.

GREEN PEA AND LEEK PUREE

Yield: 4 to 6 servings
Soundtrack: "Hussel" by M.I.A. featuring Afrikan Boy from *Kala*

My little cousin called this dish green mashed potatoes. Similar to mashed potatoes this dish makes a tasty side, but it is less starchy. It is high in vitamins A and B and contains lots of calcium and potassium.

Coarse sea salt

1 1/2 cups cleaned (page 99) and thinly sliced leeks (white and tender green parts)

2 1/4 pounds green peas in pod (will yield about 3 cups peas), shelled (3 cups frozen can work)

2 tablespoons extra-virgin olive oil

Freshly ground black pepper

- Bring 3 quarts of water to a boil in a large pot over high heat and add 1 tablespoon of salt. Add the leeks and the green peas, bring back to a boil, and cook, uncovered, for 3 minutes, until softened.
- Remove 6 tablespoons of the cooking liquid, add it to a small bowl, and set aside.
- Drain the leeks and peas in a colander, and transfer them to an upright blender. Add the olive oil, 1/2 teaspoon of salt, and 6 tablespoons of the reserved cooking liquid. Process until creamy, scraping down the sides of the blender and whipping a few times with a wooden spoon.
- Season with salt and pepper to taste, and serve hot.

SAUTÉED JALAPEÑO CORN

Yield: 4 to 6 servings

Soundtrack: "Imagino Como Sera" by Ceci Bastida featuring Rakaa Iriscience from *Veo La Marea*

As a part of the seminal "Slow Food Nation" held in San Francisco in the summer of 2008, I did a cooking demonstration in the Green Kitchen, where Alice Waters invited chefs to conduct short cooking demonstrations. When she asked me what ingredient I wanted to work with in order to illustrate "the basics of preparing simple, artful, sustainable food," without even thinking I said "fresh sweet corn." I created this dish to share that day.

Coarse sea salt

3 cups fresh sweet corn, from about 6 ears

1 tablespoon extra-virgin olive oil

1 clove garlic, minced

1/2 teaspoon ground cumin

2 jalapeños, seeded and minced

Freshly ground white pepper

- Bring 2 quarts of water to a boil in a medium pot over high heat and add 2 teaspoons of salt. Add the corn, immediately remove from heat, and let sit for 30 seconds. Drain in a colander.

- In a medium-size sauté pan over medium heat, combine the olive oil, garlic, cumin, and 1/4 teaspoon of salt and sauté, stirring often, until fragrant, about 2 minutes.

- Add the corn and jalapeño and cook, stirring frequently, until thoroughly mixed, 3 to 5 minutes.

- Season with salt and white pepper to taste.

SWEET COCONUT-GINGER CREAMED CORN

Yield: 4 to 6 servings
Soundtrack: "Duppy Conqueror" by Bob Marley & The Wailers from *African Herbsman*

I originally made this dish to be used as a filling for **Jamaican Veggie Patties** (page 111), but I most often have this as a side dish sans the pastry (although you should feel free to use it as a filling for the patties). Reminds me of the creamed corn that mom used to make when I was growing up.

1 tablespoon coconut oil

1 small red onion, cut into 1/4-inch dice

1/2 teaspoon ground allspice

Coarse sea salt

3 cups fresh sweet corn, from about 6 ears

1 tablespoon minced fresh ginger

1 cup coconut milk

1 teaspoon organic raw cane sugar

Freshly ground white pepper

- In a medium-size sauté pan over low heat, combine coconut oil, onion, allspice, and 1/8 teaspoon salt and sauté, stirring often, until caramelized, 10 to 12 minutes.
- Add the corn and the ginger, raise the heat to medium, and cook, stirring frequently, until soft, about 5 minutes.
- Reduce the heat to low, add the coconut milk and the sugar and simmer, stirring often, for 10 minutes.
- Season with salt and white pepper to taste.

CRISP GREEN BEANS WITH ROASTED SHALLOTS AND WALNUTS

Yield: 4 to 6 servings

Soundtrack: "Down Here on the Ground" by Grant Green from *Alive!*

Art: "16 cowries/seeds" by Eesuu Orundide

Coarse sea salt

1 pound fresh green beans, snapped at each end

1/4 cup freshly squeezed lemon juice

2 tablespoons red wine vinegar

2 teaspoons Dijon mustard

2 teaspoons agave nectar or pure maple syrup

2 large cloves garlic, minced

1 tablespoon fresh thyme

1/2 cup plus 1 teaspoon extra-virgin olive oil

Freshly ground white pepper

4 large shallots

1/4 cup walnut halves, toasted, skins removed and coarsely chopped (page 40)

- Bring 4 quarts of water to a boil in a large pot over high heat and add 1 tablespoon of salt. Add the green beans and cook 4 to 5 minutes, until tender but still al dente. Drain the beans into a colander and shock in a bowl filled with ice water to stop cooking. Drain again and place in a large serving bowl.

- In a blender, combine the lemon juice, vinegar, mustard, agave nectar, garlic, thyme, and 3/4 teaspoon salt. Slowly pour in 1/2 cup of olive oil with the blender going. Add white pepper to taste.

- Toss the green beans with the vinaigrette to coat well and set aside.

- Preheat oven to 425°F.

- In a small bowl, toss the shallots with 1 teaspoon of olive oil and 1/4 teaspoon of salt.

- Transfer to a parchment-lined baking sheet and bake until the shallots are charred on the outside and tender on the inside. Remove from the oven and allow to cool. Cut off and discard the blossom ends of the shallots, squeeze the shallots from their skins, and cut them into 1/2-inch pieces.

- Add the shallots and the walnuts to the green beans. Toss well, and immediately remove all the ingredients with a slotted spoon to a serving bowl. Season with white pepper to taste.

FRIED GREEN TOMATOES WITH CREAMY CELERIAC SAUCE

Yield: 4 servings
Soundtrack: "Lay My Burden Down" by Margaret Allison & The Angelic Gospel Singers from *I've Weathered the Storm*

This Southern classic makes a tasty side dish or a light meal with a salad.

----

4 large firm green tomatoes

Coarse sea salt

1/2 cup apple cider vinegar

1/2 cup extra-virgin olive oil plus more as needed

1 cup of **Multipurpose Coating for Dredging Foods** (page 167)

Creamy Celeriac Sauce (page 170)

- Preheat the oven to 200°F.
- With a serrated knife, remove the stem and blossom ends from the tomatoes. Slice each tomato lengthwise from stem to blossom end into 1/4-inch slices and place on a large serving platter or plate in one layer.
- Lightly sprinkle with salt and set aside for 10 minutes.
- Pour the vinegar into a small bowl and spread the Multipurpose Coating for Dredging Foods on a large plate.
- One at a time, dip the tomato slices into the vinegar, then coat with the Multipurpose Coating, then dip back into the vinegar, and then coat with the Multipurpose Coating again. Shake off the excess and transfer back to the serving platter. Repeat until all the tomatoes are coated.
- In a wide, heavy sauté pan over medium-high heat, warm the oil until it is hot enough to fry a piece of Multipurpose Coating dropped in it.
- With a metal spatula, transfer as many tomatoes slices as will fit comfortably in the pan and fry until crisp and golden brown, about 1 minute on each side. Transfer the fried tomatoes to a paper towel–lined plate and allow them to drain, about 30 seconds on each side. Transfer the drained tomato slices to the baking sheet and hold in the oven to keep warm.
- Repeat with the remaining tomato slices, adding oil as necessary.
- Serve hot with the Creamy Celeriac Sauce.

JAMAICAN VEGGIE PATTIES

Yield: 6 servings
Soundtrack: "Ghetto Youth" by Tricky from *Pre-Millennium Tension*
Film: *Life and Debt* (2001), directed by Stephanie Black. This documentary explores economic globalization and its impact on the Jamaican economy.

I had to take it back to Brooklyn.

From the time I moved there until the year I moved to Oakland, veggie patties were one of my staples. I lived in Crown Heights my first year, and there was a slammin' Jamaican restaurant right down the block from my apartment. One of those hole-in-the-wall joints that always had a line extending to the sidewalk. When I moved to Clinton Hill there was a Golden Crust Restaurant around the corner from my spot that always held it down (but not as good as the first place). I know they are often eaten as a snack, but when you're living on a graduate school stipend of $15,000 per year in New York City, a $1.50 veggie pattie moves quickly into the meal column. I do the same with these, usually eating them with a large green salad. You can also use **Sweet Coconut-Ginger Creamed Corn** (page 108) as their filling.

Filling

1 tablespoon coconut oil
1/2 cup 1/4-inch-diced yellow onion
1/8 teaspoon ground cinnamon
1/4 teaspoon ground allspice
1/2 teaspoon ground cumin
1/4 teaspoon red pepper flakes
1/8 teaspoon cayenne
Coarse sea salt
2 large cloves garlic, minced
3/4 cup coconut milk
1/4 cup 1/4-inch-diced carrots
1/4 cup 1/4-inch-diced yellow potatoes
1/2 cup fresh green peas, rinsed
    (use frozen if fresh are unavailable)
1/2 cup fresh sweet corn (you can also
    use frozen if fresh isn't available)
1/2 cup shredded cabbage
1 tablespoon minced fresh thyme
1 tablespoon freshly squeezed
    lemon juice
1/2 teaspoon freshly ground white
    pepper

Pastry

1 3/4 cups unbleached white flour, chilled
1 cup whole wheat pastry flour, chilled
2 teaspoons turmeric
1/2 teaspoon fine sea salt
3/4 cup chilled coconut butter
2 teaspoons apple cider vinegar
1/2 cup plus 2 tablespoons ice water

For the filling

- In a medium-size sauté pan over medium-low heat, combine the coconut oil, the onion, cinnamon, allspice, cumin, red pepper flakes, cayenne, and 1/2 teaspoon salt. Sauté, stirring occasionally, for 8 to 10 minutes, or until the vegetables are caramelized. Add the garlic and cook for an additional 2 minutes. Stir in the coconut milk, carrots, and potatoes, reduce the heat to low, cover, and cook until the carrots and potatoes are tender, 10 to 12 minutes. Stir in the green peas, corn, cabbage, thyme, and lemon juice, cover, and cook for 3 minutes more.
- Season with additional salt and pepper to taste and set aside to allow the flavors to marry.

For the pastry

- Combine 1 1/2 cups of the white flour with the pastry flour, turmeric, and salt in a large bowl and mix well. Set the remaining 1/4 cup white flour aside. Add the coconut butter to the flour mixture and rub with your fingertips until the mixture resembles fine sand, about 10 minutes.
- Combine the vinegar and water and mix well. Then, without overworking the dough, add the vinegar mixture by the tablespoon, while stirring, just until the dough comes away from the sides of the bowl and starts to coalesce. Squeeze into a tight ball, flatten, cover in plastic wrap, and refrigerate for at least 1 hour.
- Preheat the oven to 350°F and remove the dough from the refrigerator.
- With the reserved flour, lightly dust a clean surface, roll out the dough until it is about 1/8 inch thick. Cut six 6-inch circles from the dough (I use a bowl). Spoon 2 heaping tablespoons of the filling onto the center of one side of each circle, leaving about a 1/8-inch border. Fold the other half over to make a half-moon, press to seal, and make ridges around the edge using a fork.
- Transfer the patties to a parchment-lined baking sheet and bake until golden brown, about 35 minutes. Serve immediately with some hot sauce.

ROASTED ROOT VEGETABLES WITH ROASTED GARLIC–LIME DIPPING SAUCE

Yield: 4 to 6 servings

Soundtrack: "Freedom" by Horace Handy from *Natty Dread a Weh She Want*

One of the ways that I get the most out of root vegetables during the winter months is by roasting, which brings out their natural sweetness and gives them a deeper, richer flavor. Feel free to substitute your favorite root vegetables in this recipe.

1/2 pound carrots, peeled and cut into 1/2-inch chunks

1/2 pound celery root peeled and cut into 1/2-inch chunks

1/2 pound parsnips, peeled and cut into 1/2-inch chunks

1/2 pound rutabaga, peeled and cut into 1/2-inch chunks

1/2 pound sweet potatoes, peeled and cut into 1/2-inch chunks

1/2 pound turnips, peeled and cut into 1/2-inch chunks

3 tablespoons extra-virgin olive oil

1/2 teaspoon coarse sea salt

Roasted Garlic–Lime Dipping Sauce (page 45)

- Preheat oven to 450°F.
- In a large bowl, combine the vegetables, the olive oil, and the salt.
- Transfer the vegetables to a large roasting pan and roast for 1 hour, stirring every 15 minutes for even cooking.
- Transfer the roasted vegetables to a large bowl and toss them in 1/2 of the Roasted Garlic–Lime Dipping Sauce.

ROASTED SWEET POTATO PUREE WITH COCONUT MILK

Yield: 4 to 6 servings

Soundtrack: "I Was the One" by Renée Wilson from *Formosa's Edge*

This dish tastes like creamy orange bliss.

----

4 pounds sweet potatoes, peeled and
    cut into 1-inch chunks

4 tablespoons agave nectar

6 tablespoons coconut oil

1/2 teaspoon coarse sea salt

1/2 cup canned coconut milk, warmed,
    plus more as needed

- Preheat oven to 400°F.
- In a large bowl, combine the sweet potatoes, agave nectar, coconut oil, and sea salt. Toss well.
- Transfer the sweet potatoes to a parchment-lined baking dish or roasting pan and roast for 40 minutes, stirring every 10 minutes.
- Remove from oven.
- In a food processor fitted with a metal blade, combine the sweet potatoes with 1/2 cup of warmed coconut milk. Puree, adding additional coconut milk for your desired consistency, and transfer to a serving dish.

CUMIN-CAYENNE MASHED POTATOES WITH CARAMELIZED ONIONS

Yield: 4 to 6 servings

Soundtrack: "Push It Along" by A Tribe Called Quest from *Peoples' Instinctive Travels & the Paths of Rhythm* and "Move" by Q-Tip from *The Renaissance*

Book: *Ida: A Sword among Lions: Ida B. Wells and the Campaign against Lynching,* by Paula J. Giddings (Amistad, 2008).

These mashed potatoes are deliciously rich, creamy, and spicy and they work well as a side to simple mains like **Rosemary-Roasted Tofu Cubes** (page 146).

- -

2 pounds Yukon Gold potatoes, peeled and cut into 1/2-inch chunks

5 tablespoons extra-virgin olive oil

1 large onion, cut into 1/4-inch dice

2 tablespoons ground cumin

1/4 teaspoon cayenne

Coarse sea salt

1/2 cup unflavored rice milk

2 tablespoons minced fresh thyme

Freshly ground white pepper

- -

- In a large pot over high heat, combine the potatoes with cold water to cover by a few inches. Bring to a rolling boil and cook until the potatoes can be easily pierced with a fork, about 25 minutes.

- While the potatoes are boiling, combine the olive oil, onion, cumin, cayenne, and 1/2 teaspoon salt in a medium-size sauté pan over low heat and sauté, stirring often, until well caramelized, about 30 minutes. Set aside.

- Remove the potatoes from the heat and drain. Return them to the pot and place on the stove.

- Combine the reserved onion mixture with the rice milk and thyme in a small saucepan over low heat and warm.

- Meanwhile, mash the potatoes well with a potato masher, fork, or the like.

- While whipping the potatoes with a wire whisk or a wooden spoon, pour in the rice milk mixture. Continue whipping until light and fluffy, about 1 minute. Season with salt and white pepper to taste and serve immediately.

LITTLE POTATO AND SWEET POTATO PANCAKES

Yield: 4 to 6 servings (10 to 12 pancakes)
Soundtrack: *We Insist!—Max Roach's Freedom Now Suite* by Abbey Lincoln & Max Roach

The delectable potato latkes served at Saul's Restaurant & Delicatessen in Berkeley inspired this dish. I had considered only using sweet potatoes, but the sweetness was a bit much. The Yukon Golds provides the perfect balance. Serve these with applesauce.

¼ banana, chopped

3 tablespoons unflavored rice milk

¾ pound Yukon Gold potatoes, peeled and coarsely grated

¾ pound sweet potatoes, peeled and coarsely grated

¼ cup grated red onion

3 tablespoons whole wheat pastry flour

1 teaspoon baking powder

½ teaspoon coarse sea salt

¼ teaspoon freshly ground white pepper

Extra-virgin olive oil

- In a blender, puree the banana in the rice milk. Set aside.
- Preheat the oven to 200°F.
- In a large bowl, combine the Yukon Gold potatoes, sweet potatoes, and onions and mix well. Drain the potatoes and onions by wrapping them in a clean dishtowel and wringing out excess liquid.
- In a large bowl, combine the potatoes, onions, flour, baking powder, salt, pepper, and the banana–rice milk mixture.
- In a large, nonstick skillet over medium heat, warm 3 tablespoons olive oil. In batches of four, spoon two tablespoons of the potato mixture into the oil and flatten with a slotted spatula. Cook until brown on the bottom. Turn and brown the second side until crisp, 3 to 5 minutes each side. Transfer the pancakes with a spatula to a paper towel–lined plate and drain. Repeat with the remaining potato mixture, adding more oil as necessary.
- After draining, keep pancakes warm in the oven.

CANDIED SWEET POTATO DISCS AND APPLE SLICES

Yield: 4 servings
Soundtrack: "Goin' to Kansas City" by Memphis Slim from *Blue This Evening*

Roasting these sweet potatoes before "candying" them helps bring out the natural sugar and allows you to use less added sweetener. The varying shapes of the discs makes for a beautiful presentation.

- -

3 large sweet potatoes (about 2½ pounds total), peeled and cut into ½-inch rounds

2 tablespoons extra-virgin olive oil

2 Golden Delicious apples, cored, peeled, and cut into ½-inch widthwise slices

1 teaspoon ground cinnamon

¼ teaspoon freshly grated nutmeg

¼ cup plus 1 tablespoon agave nectar

½ teaspoon vanilla extract

2 teaspoons freshly squeezed lemon juice

½ cup freshly squeezed orange juice

¼ cup cold apple juice

½ teaspoon coarse sea salt

- -

- Preheat the oven to 425°F.

- In a large bowl, toss the sweet potatoes with 1 tablespoon of the olive oil.

- Spread the sweet potatoes on a parchment-lined baking sheet in a single layer and roast for 40 minutes, turning the discs over with a fork after 20 minutes.

- Remove the sweet potatoes from the oven and reduce the heat to 375°F.

- In a 2-quart baking dish, add a layer of sweet potatoes to the bottom, layer half of the apple slices on top of the first layer, layer the remaining sweet potatoes on top of the apples, and layer the remaining apples on top.

- In a medium-size bowl, combine 2 tablespoons of the apple juice with the cinnamon and nutmeg and mix well until the spices are evenly distributed. Add the agave nectar, vanilla extract, lemon juice, orange juice, apple juice, and salt and mix well to combine. Pour over the sweet potatoes and apples.

- Bake uncovered, for 40 minutes, basting every 10 minutes.

COLLARD CONFETTI

Yield: depends on how many stems you cook

Soundtrack: "Bits and Pieces" by Joan Jett & The Blackhearts from *I Love Rock-n-Roll*

While many people discard the stems (or ribs) of leafy greens, I often cut them into small pieces and cook them along with their leaves or incorporate them into stir-fries to add more texture. I also prepare the stems separately and make nutrient-dense confetti-like dishes to be served as a green side. I lean toward collard stems because they tend to be thick and more substantial than others, but you can use the ribs of any leafy greens for this recipe. It is written for the stems from a typical half-pound bunch of collard greens, so adjust accordingly to suit your amount.

---

1 teaspoon extra-virgin olive oil

Stems from leafy greens, thinly sliced

Coarse sea salt

2 teaspoons freshly squeezed lemon juice

Freshly ground white pepper

- In a large sauté pan over medium-high heat, warm the olive oil. Add the stems and 1/4 teaspoon of salt. Sauté for 2 to 3 minutes, stirring often, until softened. Add the lemon juice and season with white pepper to taste.

SPICY SMOTHERED GREEN CABBAGE

Yield: 4 to 6 servings
Soundtrack: "Chicken Grease" by
D'Angelo from *Voodoo*

Rather than frying this cabbage in bacon
fat, I add mustard seeds, red pepper flakes,
and sugar to the olive oil to add flavor.

2 tablespoons extra-virgin olive oil

2 teaspoons mustard seeds

1/4 to 1/2 teaspoon red pepper flakes

1 teaspoon organic raw cane sugar

Coarse sea salt

1 small green cabbage (about 2 pounds),
   quartered, cored, and sliced thinly

5 tablespoons water

Freshly ground white pepper

- In a wide, heavy sauté pan over medium heat, combine the olive oil, mustard seeds, red pepper flakes, sugar, and 1/2 teaspoon sea salt. Cook, stirring frequently, until the mustard seeds start to pop, about 2 minutes.
- Immediately add the cabbage and sauté, stirring occasionally, until it wilts, about 4 minutes.
- Add the water, stir to combine, cover, and cook until most of the water has evaporated, about 4 minutes.
- Season with white pepper to taste.

WILTED SWISS CHARD AND SPINACH WITH LEMON-TAHINI DRESSING

Yield: 4 to 6 servings
Soundtrack: "Black History Month" by Saul Williams from *The Inevitable Rise and Liberation of Niggy Tardust!*

I add bright red chard to give this dish color. Leaving on the spines adds more texture, but feel free to remove them.

Lemon-Tahini Dressing

½ cup tahini

¼ cup water

¼ cup freshly squeezed lemon juice

2 teaspoons balsamic vinegar

3 cloves garlic, minced

½ teaspoon coarse sea salt

Chard and Spinach

8 packed cups chopped red chard (others can be used), cut into bite-size pieces

8 packed cups chopped spinach leaves, cut into bite-size pieces

---

For the dressing

- Combine all the ingredients in an upright blender and blend until creamy.

For the chard and spinach

- In a large sauté pan over medium heat, cook the chard and spinach down, stirring often, about 5 minutes.
- Transfer to a colander and drain.
- Combine the wilted chard and spinach with enough dressing to coat lightly and toss well.

GARLIC BROTH–BRAISED BRUSSELS SPROUTS

Yield: 4 servings
Soundtrack: "I'm a Man" by Bo Diddley from *I'm a Man—The Chess Masters, 1955–1958*

I'm always trying to help people recover from Brussels sprouts trauma and get them to appreciate how tasty baby cabbages can be. As long as they are not boiled to death, you should be okay. Braising them in garlic broth until meltingly tender makes them less bitter and deeply flavorful.

2 tablespoons extra-virgin olive oil

1 pound Brussels sprouts, trimmed of stems and cut in half lengthwise

1 cup **Garlic Broth** (page 77)

Coarse sea salt

¼ cup white wine

2 tablespoons minced fresh thyme

White pepper

- Coat a large sauté pan with the olive oil. Add the Brussels sprouts, arranging them cut side down, making one snug layer. Turn the heat to medium-high and sauté until the cut sides are lightly browned, 2 to 3 minutes.
- Add the Garlic Broth and 1 teaspoon sea salt. Bring to a boil and stir well. Immediately reduce the temperature to low, cover tightly, and braise for 15 minutes. Add the white wine and the thyme, stir well, cover, and braise 5 minutes more, until the Brussels sprouts are meltingly tender.
- Remove from the heat.
- Season with additional salt and pepper to taste and serve hot.

ROASTED POTATO AND MIXED GREENS GRATIN

Yield: 4 to 6 servings
Soundtrack: "Give Me a Chance" by
Sharon Jones & The Dap-Kings from
*Dap-Dippin' with Sharon Jones and
The Dap Kings*

Roasted potatoes provide a starchy
contrast to each greens-packed bite of this
gratin. The crispy bread crumbs add more
texture.

3 to 4 medium yellow potatoes
(about 1¼ pounds), peeled and
sliced into ¼-inch rounds

6 tablespoons extra-virgin olive oil plus
more for oiling the baking dish

½ teaspoon chili powder

½ teaspoon crushed red pepper flakes

½ teaspoon dried thyme

½ teaspoon dried oregano

Coarse sea salt

1 bunch collard greens (about 1 pound),
trimmed and chopped into bite-size
pieces

1 bunch mustard greens (about 1 pound),
trimmed and chopped into bite-size
pieces

4 large cloves garlic, minced

1 cup panko bread crumbs

1½ cups unflavored rice milk

Freshly ground white pepper

- Preheat the oven to 450°F.
- In a large bowl, toss the potatoes with
  1 tablespoon olive oil, the chili powder,
  red pepper flakes, thyme, oregano, and
  ¼ teaspoon salt.
- Transfer the potatoes to a parchment-lined
  baking sheet, spread in one layer, and
  roast for 20 minutes. Gently turn the potatoes over with a fork and roast for another
  15 to 20 minutes, or until the potatoes are
  tender and browned.
- Remove the potatoes from the oven and
  reduce the heat to 350°F.

- While the potatoes are roasting, bring 4 quarts of water to a boil in a large pot. Add 2 teaspoons of salt and the greens and cook, uncovered, for 5 minutes, until shrunk down. Drain in a colander.
- In a heavy, wide sauté pan, combine 2 tablespoons of olive oil and the garlic. Turn the heat to medium and sauté until fragrant, about 1 minute. Add the greens and 1/2 teaspoon salt, raise the heat to high, and sauté, stirring often, until the greens are well coated with oil and most of the liquid has evaporated, about 2 minutes. Remove from heat.
- Transfer the greens to a colander and press them gently to extract their excess liquid. Remove to a cutting board and coarsely chop.
- In a small bowl, combine the bread crumbs with 3 tablespoons of olive oil.
- Lightly oil a casserole dish. Arrange one layer of the potatoes on the bottom. Spread half of the greens over the potatoes and repeat the layer. Pour the rice milk over the top over the gratin. Spread the bread crumbs evenly on top of the gratin, cover with aluminum foil, and bake for 45 minutes.
- Remove the foil and place under the broiler for a few minutes to brown the top.
- Add pepper to taste and serve immediately.

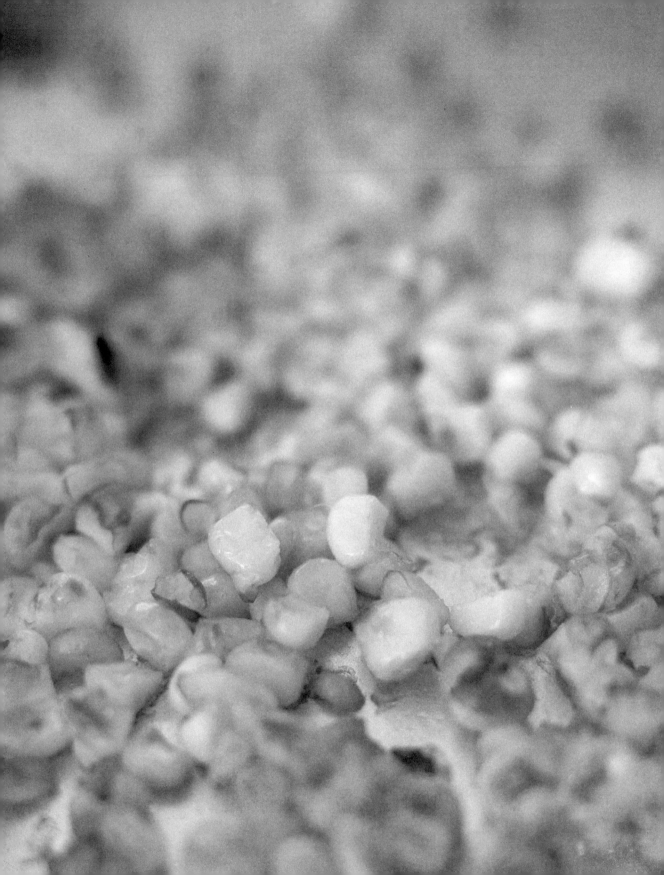

BRING THE GRAIN
RICE. OATS. ANCIENT GRAINS. GRITS.

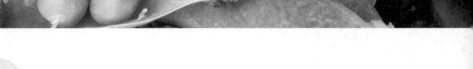

- Brown Coconut Rice •

• New World Red Rice •

• Not-Too-Dirty Rice •

• Maple-Almond Granola •

• Black. Brown. Green. Granola. •

• Brown Steel (Cut Oats) in the Hour of Quiescence •

• Power Porridge •

• Savory Triple-Corn Grits •

• Upper Caribbean Creamy Grits with
Roasted Plantain Pieces •

• Pan-Fried Grit Cakes with Caramelized
Spring Onions, Garlic, and Thyme •

Rice

BROWN COCONUT RICE

Yield: 4 to 6 servings

Soundtrack: "Hi Sun" by J*Davey from *The Land of the Lost*

The coconut milk gives this rice a rich flavor and provides an alternative to plain brown rice.

1 cup short-grain brown rice

¾ cup coconut milk

1½ cups water

Coarse sea salt

3 tablespoons unsweetened shredded coconut

- Add the rice to a medium bowl, cover with at least 2½ cups water, and refrigerate overnight.
- Drain the rice into a colander and set aside.
- In a medium-size saucepan over high heat, combine the coconut milk, 1½ cups water, and ½ teaspoon salt. Bring to a boil, add the rice and dried coconut, stir well, and bring back to a boil. Cover the pot with a lid, reduce the heat to low, and cook for 50 minutes.
- Remove from heat and steam with lid on for at least 10 minutes, then fluff with a fork before serving.

SOAKING AND COOKING RICE

Soaking rice shortens its cooking time and makes it more digestible. I usually add mine to the saucepan in which it will be cooked, cover it with the measured amount of cooking liquid (unlike with beans, you can cook rice in its soaking liquid), and soak it overnight in the refrigerator. You can also soak it at room temperature for an hour or so. Remember, when cooking rice, don't lift the lid, as this releases steam and slows down the cooking process. And unless a recipe calls for it, do not stir rice until it's done. You will disturb the steam holes and make it harder to cook. Always let your rice steam with the lid on for 5 to 10 minutes when you remove it from the heat to allow it to continue cooking.

NEW WORLD RED RICE

Yield: 4 to 6 servings
Soundtrack: "Ça Varie" by Zap Mama from *Ancestry in Progress*
Art: "Soon Be Free" by Keba Konte

This dish is inspired by red rice, which is normally served with my favorite Senegalese dish, Thiebou Dienn—a savory rice and fish stew that is the national dish of Senegal.

1 cup short-grain brown rice, soaked in water overnight

4 tablespoons peanut oil

1 cup yellow onion, diced

½ teaspoon paprika

½ teaspoon chili powder

⅛ teaspoon cayenne

1 red jalapeño (green will work), seeded and cut into ½-inch dice

4 cloves garlic, minced

1½ cups chopped canned tomatoes with their juices

1 tablespoon tomato paste

2 tablespoons tamari

2½ cups **Simple Stock** (page 76)

2 tablespoons minced fresh thyme

- Drain the rice and set aside.
- In a medium-size saucepan over low heat, combine the peanut oil, onion, paprika, chili powder, and cayenne and sauté until well caramelized, 10 to 15 minutes. Add the rice and cook for about 2 minutes, stirring often, until the water has evaporated and the rice start to smell nutty. Add the jalapeño and garlic and cook until fragrant, about 1½ minutes.
- Stir in the tomatoes and their juices, the tomato paste, the tamari, and the Simple Stock. Bring to a boil, cover, reduce heat to low, and cook for 45 minutes.
- Remove from heat, stir in the thyme, and steam with cover on for at least 10 minutes.
- Season with additional tamari to taste and serve.

NOT-TOO-DIRTY RICE

Yield: 4 to 6 servings
Soundtrack: "Very Special" by Duke Ellington, Charlie Mingus, and Max Roach from *Money Jungle*

Dirty Rice is a traditional Cajun dish that gets its "dirtiness" from chopped-up pieces of liver. This version use seitan and tempeh instead.

- -

1 cup long-grain brown rice, soaked in
    water overnight

8 ounces seitan, chopped finely

3 tablespoons extra-virgin olive oil

1 cup diced red onion

1 cup diced green bell pepper

1 celery stalk, peeled of string fibers and
    chopped finely

1 teaspoon paprika

1/2 teaspoon chili powder

1/4 teaspoon cayenne

2 tablespoons tamari

1/4 pound tempeh (half 8-ounce
    package), crumbled

3 cloves garlic, minced

2 1/4 cups **Simple Stock** (page 76)

1/4 cup minced fresh parsley

Freshly ground white pepper

- -

- Drain the rice and set aside.

- In a clean kitchen towel or paper towels, squeeze the seitan of its moisture and set aside.

- In a medium-size saucepan over medium heat, combine the olive oil, onion, bell pepper, celery, paprika, chili powder, cayenne, and tamari and sauté, stirring often, until vegetables are soft, about 5 minutes. Add the seitan, tempeh, garlic, and reserved rice and cook until fragrant, about 3 minutes.

- Add the stock to the saucepan and stir well, scraping the bottom of the pan to release any solids. Bring to a boil, cover, reduce heat to low, and cook for 50 minutes, until most of the water has evaporated.

- Remove from heat and steam with cover on for at least 10 minutes.

- Stir in the parsley. Season with white pepper and tamari to taste and serve hot.

Oats and Ancient Grains

MAPLE-ALMOND GRANOLA

Yield: about 5 cups
Soundtrack: "What Your Soul Sings" by Massive Attack featuring Sinéad O'Connor from *100th Window*

3 cups old-fashioned rolled oats

½ cup melted coconut oil

½ cup pure maple syrup

2 cups raw almonds

- Preheat oven to 300°F.
- Evenly spread the oats on a parchment-lined baking sheet and toast for 20 minutes, stirring every 5 minutes for even toasting. Remove from the oven and transfer to a large bowl.
- In a small bowl, combine the coconut oil and maple syrup and mix well.
- Add the almonds and coconut oil mixture to the bowl with the oats and mix well with a large spoon.
- Evenly spread the granola on the baking sheet used to toast the oats and bake, stirring every 10 minutes, until well toasted and golden brown, about 45 minutes.
- After cooling, transfer to a tightly sealed container and store in the refrigerator for up to one month.

BLACK. BROWN.
GREEN. GRANOLA.

Yield: about 5 cups
Soundtrack: *Black, Brown and Beige* by
Duke Ellington featuring Mahalia Jackson
Art: "The Interaction of Coloreds" by
Mendi+Keith Obadike

I have been experimenting with granola
for a while now, and this one is not only
tasty but highly nutritious. The pumpkin
seeds are an excellent source of iron, zinc,
phosphorous, Vitamin A, calcium, and Vitamin B. I serve mine with almost-frozen
Almond Milk (page 28).

- -

4 cups old-fashioned rolled oats

1½ cups raw pumpkin seeds

¾ cup unsweetened shredded coconut

¼ teaspoon fine sea salt

2 teaspoons ground cinnamon

½ cup apple cider

½ cup melted coconut oil

½ cup pure maple syrup

2 teaspoons vanilla extract

1 cup chopped dried black mission figs,
   tough tips discarded

½ cup currants

- -

- Preheat oven to 350°F.
- Evenly spread the oats on a parchment-lined baking sheet and toast for 20 minutes, stirring every 5 minutes for even toasting. Remove from the oven and transfer to a large bowl.
- Reduce the oven's temperature to 325°F.
- Add the pumpkin seeds, shredded coconut, salt, and cinnamon to the bowl with the oats and mix well with a large spoon.
- In a medium-size bowl, combine the apple cider, coconut oil, maple syrup, and vanilla extract and mix well. Transfer to the bowl with the oats mixture and stir to combine until well coated.
- Evenly spread the granola on the baking sheet used to toast the oats and bake, stirring every 10 minutes, until well toasted and golden brown, about 45 minutes.
- While the granola is toasting, combine the figs and currants in a small bowl and cover with boiling water for 1 minute to reconstitute. Drain and set aside.
- Remove the granola from the oven, transfer to a large bowl, stir in the reconstituted figs and currants, and transfer back to the baking sheet to cool.
- After cooling, transfer to a tightly sealed container and store in the refrigerator for up to one month.

BROWN STEEL (CUT OATS) IN THE HOUR OF QUIESCENCE

Yield: 4 to 6 servings

Soundtrack: "Black Steel in the Hour of Chaos" by Public Enemy from *It Takes a Nation of Millions to Hold Us Back* and "Black Steel" by Tricky from *Maxinquaye*

When I was growing up I suffered through bowls of thirsty-for-more-liquid instant rolled oats for too many breakfasts. As an adult, I gained an appreciation for their far more superior cousin—steel-cut oats (also known as Scottish or Irish oats). These days, I turn to lighter breakfast fare during the warmer months. But in the late fall, winter, and early spring I'm all about porridges, and steel-cut oats are often one of the main ingredients. Here is a simple and hearty breakfast porridge that helps me start my day off right. Feel free to add more fresh or dried fruit.

---

1 teaspoon ground cinnamon

1 cup plus 1 tablespoon water

1 cup steel-cut oats

3 cups **Almond Milk** (page 28) or unflavored rice milk

Fine sea salt

½ teaspoon coconut oil

½ cup currants

1 cup pecan halves, toasted and half of them chopped (page 41)

2 tablespoons pure maple syrup

- In a small bowl, combine the cinnamon with 1 tablespoon of water and mix until well combined. In a medium-size saucepan, combine the cinnamon-water slurry, the remaining water, the oats, the Almond Milk, and ¼ teaspoon salt. Swish around, cover, and refrigerate at least 6 hours, or overnight.

- Over medium heat bring the oats to a boil. Add the coconut oil and cook, stirring constantly, until they start to thicken, about 2 to 3 minutes. Immediately reduce the heat to low, and simmer, uncovered, for 20 minutes, stirring often to prevent from sticking to the bottom of the pan.

- Add the currants and simmer for an additional 5 minutes. Remove from heat, stir in the pecans and maple syrup, let stand for 5 minutes, and serve.

POWER PORRIDGE

Yield: 4 to 6 servings

Soundtrack: "Maria Lando" by Susana Baca from *The Soul of Black Peru—Afro-Peruvian Classics,* "Brown Paper People" by Lila Downs from *One Blood—Una Sangre,* and "Angelitos Negros" by Roberta Flack from *First Take*

Art: "El Negro Mas Chulo: African by Legacy, Mexican by Birth": photography series by Ayana Vellissia Jackson and Marcos Villalobos and "Exile on Main Street (*laberinto de espejos y transformacion*)" by William Cordova

Talk about power . . . amaranth and quinoa are both high in protein, contain more calcium than milk, and are great sources of dietary fiber and minerals. Considered sacred thousands of years ago by the Aztecs (amaranth) and Incas (quinoa), these grains were the center of ceremonial rituals before Spanish colonizers forbade their cultivation. Over the last thirty years they have regained popularity as "superfoods."

In addition to introducing you to one of my favorite porridges that uses both of these ancient grains, I wanted an opportunity to bring up the oft-overlooked African presence in contemporary Mexico and South America that began when the conquistadors brought enslaved Africans with them to serve as laborers. I dedicate this dish to all those who have historically dealt with the negative effects of colonialism, industrialization, and the "spreading of democracy."

½ cup water

2 cups **Almond Milk** (page 28) or unflavored rice milk, plus more for creaminess

1 cinnamon stick

½ cup quinoa, rinsed

½ cup amaranth

¼ teaspoon coarse sea salt

½ teaspoon coconut oil

1 cup banana chips

¼ cup Thompson raisins

1 tablespoon flaxseed powder

2 teaspoons agave nectar

- In a medium-size saucepan over medium heat, combine the water, Almond Milk, cinnamon stick, quinoa, amaranth, salt, and coconut oil. Bring to a boil, and quickly reduce the heat to low. Cover and simmer for 20 minutes.
- Add the banana chips, raisins, flaxseed powder, and agave nectar, and stir to incorporate. Add more rice milk to your desired creaminess.
- Remove from heat, let stand for 5 minutes, and serve.

Grits

SAVORY TRIPLE-CORN GRITS

Yield: 4 to 6 servings
Soundtrack: "Smash on tha System" by
Ras K'dee from *Street Prison*

Peter Berley's Triple-Corn Polenta with
Seaweed and Carrots from his book *The
Modern Vegetarian Kitchen* inspired this
recipe.

2 large ears fresh sweet corn, kernels
   scraped

2 tablespoons extra-virgin olive oil

1 large onion, diced

1 teaspoon ground cumin

Coarse sea salt

2 cloves garlic, minced

½ cup cornmeal

½ cup stone-ground grits

4 cups water

½ cup **Creamed Cashews** (page 168)

Freshly ground white pepper

- Bring a large pot of salted water to a boil.
  Turn off the heat, add the corn, and let sit
  for 1 minute. Drain and set aside.

- In a medium-size sauté pan over medium
  heat, warm the olive oil and add the onion,
  cumin, and ½ teaspoon salt. Cook for
  about 7 minutes, stirring occasionally, until
  softened. Add the garlic and cook for 2
  minutes more, or until the garlic has softened. Remove half of the onion mixture to
  a small bowl and set aside. Add the reserved corn and cook for an additional
  2 minutes. Set aside.

- In a bowl, combine the cornmeal and grits
  and mix well. In a medium-size saucepan,
  combine 3 cups of the water and ½ teaspoon of salt and bring to a boil. Whisk the
  cornmeal and grits into the liquid until no
  lumps remain, return to a boil, then quickly
  reduce the heat to low, and simmer, stirring occasionally to prevent the grits from
  sticking to the bottom of the pan, until the
  grits have absorbed most of the liquid and
  are thickening, about 3 minutes. Stir in the
  remaining cup of water and simmer for another 10 minutes, stirring occasionally, until most of the liquid has been absorbed.
  Stir in the Creamed Cashews and the corn
  mixture, cover, and simmer, stirring frequently, until the grits are soft and fluffy,
  about 30 minutes.

- Season with salt and white pepper to
  taste. Garnish each serving with some of
  the reserved onion mixture.

UPPER CARIBBEAN CREAMY GRITS WITH ROASTED PLANTAIN PIECES

Yield: 4 to 6 servings
Soundtrack: "Tie My Hands" by
Lil Wayne from *Tha Carter III*
Art: "The Block" by Terrance Osborne

I originally made these grits to be paired with my **Cajun-Creole-Spiced Tempeh Pieces with Creamy Grits** (page 10), but the coconut milk made the grits sweeter than I wanted them to be for that dish. So I decided to add some cinnamon, ginger, and a dollop of maple syrup and make this a breakfast dish.

---

1 large ripe yellow plantain, ends cut off, peeled, cut in half lengthwise and cut into 1/2-inch pieces widthwise

1 teaspoon extra-virgin olive oil

1/2 teaspoon ground cinnamon

Coarse sea salt

1 1/2 cups coconut milk

1 tablespoon minced ginger

1 cinnamon stick

4 cups water

3/4 cup stone-ground grits

5 tablespoons maple crystals or organic raw cane sugar

- Preheat oven to 450°F.

- In a small bowl, toss the plantains, olive oil, cinnamon, and 1/8 teaspoon salt. Transfer to a parchment-lined baking sheet and cook, stirring a few times to ensure even browning, until crisp on the outside and starting to turn golden brown, about 45 minutes. Set aside.

- In a small saucepan over medium-low heat, combine the coconut milk, the ginger, and the cinnamon stick. Simmer for 5 minutes, stirring often and ensuring that the coconut milk does not boil. Remove from the heat and strain the coconut milk into a small bowl. Set aside.

- In a medium-size saucepan, combine 3 cups of the water and 1/2 teaspoon salt and bring to a boil. Whisk the grits into the liquid until no lumps remain, return to a boil, then quickly reduce the heat to medium-low, and simmer, stirring occasionally to prevent the grits from sticking to the bottom of the pan, until the grits have absorbed most of the liquid and are thickening, 10 to 12 minutes. Stir in the remaining cup of water and cook for another 10 minutes, stirring occasionally, until most of the liquid has been absorbed. Stir in the reserved coconut milk and simmer, stirring frequently, until the grits are soft but not runny, 30 to 35 minutes. Stir in the maple sugar.

- Right before serving top each serving with some roasted plantains.

PAN-FRIED GRIT CAKES WITH CARAMELIZED SPRING ONIONS, GARLIC, AND THYME

Yield: 4 to 6 servings
Soundtrack: "Green Onions" by
Booker T. & the MG's from *Green Onions*

Because the grits need to set for a few hours before you can cut them, this dish should be prepared in advance. The time invested is well worth it. I enjoy these tasty cakes as a savory dinner side or as a light meal with a green salad. You can omit the spring onions, cayenne, garlic, and thyme and reduce the salt to 1/2 teaspoon then eat these with pure maple syrup as a breakfast treat. Or you can eat them as is with maple syrup like my mom does.

For a low-fat version, they can be baked on a lightly greased baking sheet at 325°F until crisp, about 15 minutes each side. They can also be lightly brushed with olive oil and grilled for 10 minutes on each side.

Extra-virgin olive oil

1 large bunch of spring onions, trimmed and sliced thinly

1/8 teaspoon cayenne

3 cloves garlic, minced

3 cups unflavored rice milk

1 cup vegetable stock

1 cup stone-ground corn grits

1/2 teaspoon coarse sea salt

1/2 teaspoon fresh thyme

- In a medium-size nonstick sauté pan, combine 1/2 tablespoon of olive oil, the spring onions, and the cayenne. Turn the heat to medium-low and sauté gently until well caramelized, 10 to 15 minutes. Add the garlic and sauté until golden, 2 to 3 minutes. Remove from the heat and set aside.

- In a medium-size saucepan, combine the rice milk with the stock, cover, bring to a boil, and boil for about 3 minutes. Uncover and whisk the grits into the liquid until no lumps remain.

- Reduce the heat to low and simmer for 25 minutes, stirring every 2 to 3 minutes with a wooden spoon to prevent the grits from sticking to the bottom of the pan.

- Add the spring onion mixture, salt, and thyme and stir well. Cook for an additional 5 minutes, stirring from time to time.

- Pour the grits into a 2-quart rectangular baking dish or a comparable mold and spread them out with a rubber spatula (the grits should be about 1/2 inch thick). Refrigerate and allow the grits to rest until firm, about 3 hours or overnight.
- Preheat the oven to 250°F.
- Slice the grits into 2-inch squares.
- Line a couple of large plates with paper towels. In a large nonstick pan over medium-high heat, warm 1 tablespoon of olive oil. When the oil is hot, panfry the cakes for 2 to 3 minutes per side, until they are golden brown and crispy on the outside (do this in several batches to avoid overcrowding the pan). Transfer the cooked cakes from the skillet to the plates to drain, and then hold them in the oven until all the cakes are cooked.
- Serve immediately.

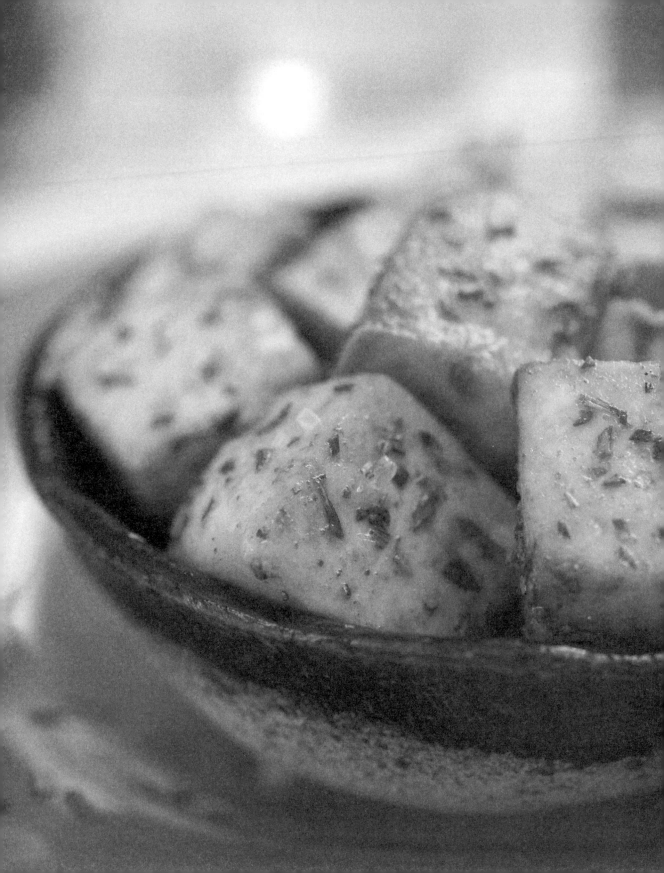

PROTEIN ROUTINE
BEANS. TOFU. TEMPEH. SEITAN.

• Creole Hoppin'-Jean [jôn] •

• Baked BBQ Black-Eyed Peas •

• Boppin' John •

• Red Beans and Brown Rice with
Red Wine–Simmered Seitan •

• Rosemary-Roasted Tofu Cubes •

• Blackened Tofu Slabs with Succotash Salsa •

• Tempeh-Stuffed Bell Peppers •

• Good Green Tempeh Packet •

• Whole-Grain Mustard and Cornmeal Crusted Seitan •

• Smothered Seitan Medallions in Mixed-Mushroom Gravy •

Beans

CREOLE HOPPIN'-JEAN [JÔN]

Yield: 4 to 6 servings
Soundtrack: "Burnin' and Lootin'" by Bob Marley from *Talkin' Blues*
Film: *La Haine* (1995), directed by Mathieu Kassovitz. This narrative film looks at the racial and cultural volatility in modern-day France.

Although Hoppin' John is mainly associated with the Carolinas, the dish is eaten throughout the South, especially on New Year's Day, when it is thought to bring the eater good luck. After returning to New Orleans from a semester abroad in France, Hoppin' John was one of the first meals that I had. Here, I reinterpret this dish adding tomatoes and a New Orleans–inspired spice blend, giving a nod to the "Afro-Euro-Creole flavors that curry favor" in Louisiana Creole cuisine, as Mike Molina would say. With all the post-Katrina politricks taking place in New Orleans the city needs all the good luck it can get.

¾ cup black-eyed peas, sorted, soaked overnight, drained, and rinsed

½ cup long-grain brown rice, rinsed and soaked overnight

1 tablespoon plus 2 teaspoons extra-virgin olive oil

½ cup finely diced shallots

⅛ teaspoon onion powder

¼ teaspoon garlic powder

½ teaspoon paprika

½ teaspoon chili powder

¼ teaspoon red pepper flakes

⅛ teaspoon cayenne

¼ teaspoon dried thyme

¼ teaspoon dried oregano

2 cups **Simple Stock** (page 76) or **'Shroom Stock** (page 79)

1 14.5-ounce can diced tomatoes, drained

1 teaspoon coarse sea salt

- Combine the black-eyed peas with enough water to cover them by 2 inches in a medium-size saucepan over high heat and bring to a boil. Skim off any foam, reduce heat to medium-low, and simmer, partially covered, just until tender, 50 minutes to 1 hour. Remove from heat and drain.

- Drain the rice and add to a medium-size saucepan. Turn the heat to medium and cook for about 2 minutes, stirring often with a wooden spoon, until the water has evaporated and the rice starts smelling nutty. Add 1 tablespoon of olive oil and continue cooking until the rice starts browning, about 2 minutes.
- Add the shallots, onion powder, garlic powder, paprika, chili powder, red pepper flakes, cayenne, thyme, oregano, and 2 teaspoons of olive oil. Continue cooking, stirring frequently, until the shallots are soft, about 3 minutes. Transfer this mixture to a bowl and set aside.
- Over medium heat in the saucepan that the rice was cooked in, combine the Simple Stock, the tomatoes, and 1 teaspoon of salt and bring to a boil. Add the rice mixture and the black-eyed peas to the stock and stir well. Bring back to a boil, then cover, reduce heat to low, and cook for 50 minutes, until most of the water has evaporated.
- Remove from heat and steam with the cover on for at least 10 minutes.
- Serve hot with your favorite hot sauce.

BEANS BASICS

Choosing

When it comes to beans and legumes I almost always choose bulk over canned (with the exception of black beans). While preparing canned beans is obviously more convenient, cooking them from scratch allows me to have control over their texture and the kind of seasonings going into them. That being said, if you are whipping up quick home meals during the week and you don't have a lot of time, it is fine to use good-quality canned beans. But I suggest starting from scratch with these recipes. And if possible, opt for bulk beans over prepackaged.

Soaking

You need to soak your dried beans before cooking them. But first you should spread them out on a baking sheet, sort through them, and pick out pebbles and other extraneous debris. Next, get rid of any shriveled or deformed beans. After rinsing the beans that you will cook a few times in cold water, place them in a pot with enough cold water to cover them by about 2 inches, so they have room to expand. Cover the pot and store them in the refrigerator overnight. Discard any beans that float to the top.

If you are in a rush, you can quick soak beans by placing them in a pot with enough cold water to cover them by about 2 inches; bringing them to a boil over high heat; covering the pot with a lid; and setting aside to soak for at least 1 hour.

Cooking

Always drain beans of their soaking water and add fresh water to cook them. Cover your beans by about 3 inches of water to ensure that they have enough room to boil. Bring them to a boil over high heat. Reduce the heat to medium, and simmer for the suggested time. Because the water will be evaporating as the beans are cooking, check them every so often in case you need to add more water. Wait until the last 10 minutes of cooking before you salt your beans, otherwise you will slow down their cooking time.

BAKED BBQ BLACK-EYED PEAS

Yield: 4 to 6 servings
Soundtrack: "Harlem" by Bill Withers
from *Just as I Am*
Art: "Portrait of James Baldwin" by
Brett Cook-Dizney
Book: *Notes of a Native Son* by
James Baldwin (Beacon Press, 1984)

This dish provides a tangy and tasty alternative to the run-of-the mill baked beans that are normally served at summer cookouts.

1½ cups dried black-eyed peas, sorted, soaked overnight, drained, and rinsed

1 3-inch piece kombu

3 tablespoons plus 2 teaspoons extra-virgin olive oil

½ cup diced onions

1 cup diced green bell pepper

2 cloves garlic, minced

2 tablespoons red wine vinegar

2 tablespoons freshly squeezed lime juice

½ cup tamari

1 cup canned tomato sauce

1 large chipotle chile in adobo sauce

¼ cup agave nectar

1 tablespoon ground cumin

Pinch of cayenne

1 teaspoon dried thyme

½ pound (1 8-ounce package) tempeh, crumbled

- Combine the black-eyed peas with the kombu and enough water to cover them by 2 inches in a medium-size saucepan over medium heat and bring to a boil. Skim off any foam, reduce the heat to medium-low, and simmer, partially covered, just until tender, 50 minutes to 1 hour. Drain the beans, reserving their cooking water.

- While the beans are cooking, combine 2 teaspoons of the olive oil, the onions, and bell pepper in a medium-size sauté pan over medium heat. Sauté for 5 to 7 minutes, or until the vegetables have softened. Add the garlic and cook for an additional 2 minutes, until fragrant.

- Preheat the oven to 350°F.

- In a blender, combine the vinegar, lime juice, tamari, tomato sauce, chile, agave nectar, cumin, cayenne, thyme, 1 cup of the reserved bean water, and the remaining olive oil. Puree for 30 seconds until smooth.

- In a cast-iron skillet or a 2-quart baking dish, combine the cooked beans with the sautéed vegetables, the tempeh, and the barbecue sauce and stir well.

- Bake, uncovered, for 2 hours, stirring occasionally.

- Serve at room temperature.

BOPPIN' JOHN

Yield: 4 to 6 servings

Soundtrack: "Koko" by Charlie "Bird" Parker from *The Complete Savoy & Dial Master Takes* and "KoKo (DJ Spooky's Ali Baba & 50 Thieves Mix)" by Charlie "Bird" Parker from *Re-Bop—The Savoy Remixes*

Yeah, I know this is the fourth recipe in this book using black-eyed peas, but I had to flip this. This remix of Hoppin' John uses **Baked BBQ Black-Eyed Peas** (page 143), and it's on hit. The plain rice is the perfect foil for the intensely flavored beans.

1/2 cup long-grain brown rice, rinsed and soaked overnight

1 cup plus 2 tablespoons water

- Drain the rice.
- In a small saucepan over high heat, combine the rice and the water, cover, and bring to a boil. Immediately reduce the heat to low and simmer for 40 minutes, until tender. Remove from heat, set aside, and let steam.
- Prepare the **Baked BBQ Black-Eyed Peas** (page 143), stirring in the reserved rice after 1 1/2 hours.
- Serve at room temperature.

RED BEANS AND BROWN RICE WITH RED WINE–SIMMERED SEITAN

Yield: 4 to 6 servings
Soundtrack: "Beans and Cornbread" by Louis Jordan & His Tympany Five from *Louis Jordan: Let the Good Times Roll—The Anthology 1938–1953*

Taking beans and rice to the next level. This dish goes nicely with the **Quinoa-Quinoa Cornbread** (page 159).

---

4 cups good-quality dry red wine

4 cloves garlic, minced and divided in half

4 tablespoons fresh thyme, minced and divided in half

2 tablespoons tamari

10 cracked black peppercorns

1 pound (16 ounces) seitan, cut into bite-size pieces

1 cup dried kidney beans, sorted, soaked overnight, drained, and rinsed

1 3-inch piece kombu

Coarse sea salt

2 tablespoons extra-virgin olive oil

1 cup finely chopped shallots

1 cup green bell pepper, cut into 1/2-inch dice

1 teaspoon red pepper flakes

2 cups cooked short-grain brown rice (page 126)

White pepper

- In a medium-size saucepan over medium-low heat, combine the wine, half of the garlic, half of the thyme, the tamari, the peppercorns, and the seitan. Simmer until the seitan has absorbed the wine's flavor, about 20 minutes. Remove from the heat, drain in a colander, and set aside.

- Combine the kidney beans and kombu with enough water to cover them by two inches in a medium-size saucepan over medium heat and bring to a boil. Skim off any foam, reduce the heat to medium-low, and simmer, partially covered, until the beans are tender but not mushy, 1 1/2 to 2 hours, adding more water as needed to keep the beans covered. Add 1 teaspoon salt for the last 10 minutes of cooking.

- While the beans are cooking, combine the olive oil, the shallots, bell pepper, red pepper flakes, and 1/4 teaspoon of salt in a medium-size sauté pan over medium heat. Sauté for 5 to 7 minutes, or until the vegetables have softened. Add the remaining garlic and cook for an additional 2 minutes, until fragrant. Set aside.

- Drain the beans, reserving 1/4 cup of the cooking liquid.

- Return the beans to the saucepan. Add rice, the remaining thyme, the reserved seitan, the cooked vegetables, the reserved cooking liquid, and 1/2 teaspoon salt. Return the saucepan to the stove and simmer over low heat, stirring well, for 5 minutes, until hot.

- Season with white pepper and additional salt to taste, and serve with your favorite hot sauce.

Tofu

ROSEMARY-ROASTED TOFU CUBES

Yield: 4 to 6 servings
Soundtrack: "Everybody Loves the Sunshine" by Roy Ayers from *Everybody Loves the Sunshine* and "Everybody Loves the Sunshine (9th Wonder Remix)" from *Verve Remixed, Vol. 4*

Crispy on the outside and creamy within, these cubes serve as a nice all-purpose protein that can be paired with more complexly flavored sides to make a complete meal.

2 pounds extra-firm tofu (2 large cakes)

2 teaspoons extra-virgin olive oil

2 tablespoons minced fresh rosemary

½ teaspoon paprika

1 teaspoon coarse sea salt

- Preheat the oven to 450°F.
- Place each tofu cake on its side and cut in half. Lay the tofu down flat, keeping the layers together, and cut it, widthwise, into three even slabs. Cut each of those slabs in half widthwise, leaving you with twelve cubes per cake (twenty-four total).
- In a medium-size bowl, combine the olive oil, rosemary, paprika, and salt and mix well with a fork. Add the tofu cubes and *gently* toss to coat with the mixture.
- *Gently* transfer the tofu cubes to a parchment-lined baking sheet in a single layer.
- Roast for 30 minutes, *gently* stirring with a large spoon after 15 minutes.

BLACKENED TOFU SLABS WITH SUCCOTASH SALSA

Yield: 4 to 6 servings
Soundtrack: "Cryin' in the Streets" by Buckwheat Zydeco from *Our New Orleans*

I substitute the succotash salsa with **Peach Salsa** (page 176) during the height of stone fruit season and eat the tofu slabs with **Brown Coconut Rice** (page 126). I also like to slice the slabs into small pieces and toss them in lettuce salads.

Salsa

5 cups water

½ cup fresh baby lima beans, rinsed (use frozen if fresh are unavailable)

1 ear sweet corn, kernels scraped

1 medium tomato, cored, seeded, and diced

3 tablespoons minced red onion

1 clove garlic, minced

1 jalapeño, seeded and chopped finely

2 tablespoons fresh cilantro, minced

1 tablespoon freshly squeezed lemon juice

¼ teaspoon coarse sea salt

Tofu Slabs

1 teaspoon onion powder

1 teaspoon garlic powder

1 tablespoon paprika

¼ teaspoon cayenne

1 tablespoon cumin

1 tablespoon coriander

1 teaspoon coarse sea salt

1 teaspoon black pepper

1 teaspoon white pepper

2 tablespoons extra-virgin olive oil

2 pounds extra-firm tofu (2 large cakes), frozen, thawed, pressed, patted dry, and (each cake) cut into 3 even, widthwise slices (sheets)

For the salsa

- In a medium-size saucepan, combine the beans with the water. Bring to a boil. Reduce the heat to medium, partially cover, and simmer for about 7 minutes, or until the beans are slightly tender. Add the corn and cook for 1 minute more. Drain.

- Plunge the beans and corn into ice water to stop the cooking and set their color. Drain.

- In a medium-size bowl, combine the lima beans, corn kernels, tomato, onion, garlic, jalapeño, cilantro, lemon juice, and salt and mix well. Set aside.

For the tofu slabs

- In a small bowl, combine the onion powder, garlic powder, paprika, cayenne, cumin, coriander, salt, black pepper, and white pepper and mix well to combine. Transfer to a large plate.

- Brush each side of the tofu sheets with olive oil, dredge with the blackened seasonings, and transfer to a plate.

- Warm a large, nonstick skillet over medium-high heat. Add the tofu to the pan and cook, without disturbing, until starting to crisp on the bottom, about 2½ minutes. With a spatula, gently turn the sheets over and fry until the other side is starting to crisp, about 2 to 3 minutes.

- Serve the salsa atop the tofu sheets with quinoa on the side.

TALKIN' TOFU

Think of tofu as a blank canvas on which you can creatively arrange colors to make a beautiful work of art. And the best way to infuse lots of flavor into tofu is to marinate it in a vegetable stock or a thin marinade by simmering it on the stovetop or baking it in the oven. Once tofu is marinated, you can take it a step further by baking, broiling, or grilling it to deepen its flavor. And if you want to add a chewy texture to tofu, I suggest freezing it for at least 24 hours (in its package) and then thawing it out in the refrigerator for 8 to 10 hours.

Before doing anything with extra-firm tofu (as opposed to silken), I suggest pressing it. This procedure extracts excess water, makes the block more uniformly firm, and allows it to absorb marinades more easily. To press a block of extra-firm tofu, wrap it in several paper towels or a clean kitchen towel, place it in a large bowl or a clean kitchen sink, and place a heavy weight on top of it for 1 hour, turning the block after 30 minutes, until most of the liquid is pressed out and absorbed by the towel.

Tempeh

TEMPEH-STUFFED BELL PEPPERS

Yield: 4 servings

Soundtrack: "Lynch Blues" by Corey Harris from *Greens from the Garden*

Film: *The Murder of Emmett Till (2003), directed by* Stanley Nelson. This documentary film tells the story of how the death of a fourteen-year-old black boy helped mobilize the civil rights movement.

Inspired by the green bell peppers that my mom used to stuff with ground beef and vegetables then top with tomato sauce, I created this version using crumbled tempeh instead. This recipe is written for four servings but there is enough filling to serve five, simply buy an additional pepper to stuff.

- -

1 cup brown basmati rice, rinsed and soaked overnight

½ cup plus 1 tablespoon extra-virgin olive oil

10 large fresh plum tomatoes

4 large red bell peppers, tops cut away and seeded

½ cup finely diced yellow onion

½ cup finely diced red onion

½ cup finely diced green bell pepper

1 pound tempeh (2 8-ounce packages), crumbled

½ teaspoon ground cumin

¼ teaspoon red pepper flakes

⅛ teaspoon cayenne

10 cloves roasted garlic

1 tablespoon red wine vinegar

¼ cup minced fresh thyme, plus more, for garnish

Freshly ground white pepper

- -

- Preheat the broiler.
- Drain the rice. In a medium-size saucepan over medium heat, sauté the rice for about 4 minutes, until the water has evaporated and the rice smells nutty, stirring well with a wooden spoon. Add 1 tablespoon of the olive oil and sauté for 1 additional minute. Add 2 cups water and bring to a boil. Cover, reduce the heat to low, and cook

- for 45 minutes, or until tender and all the water has been absorbed. Remove from the heat, let it stand with the lid on for 10 minutes, then fluff the rice with a fork. Remove the lid and set the rice aside to cool a bit.
- While the rice is cooking, place the tomatoes on a parchment-lined baking sheet. Broil fairly close to the heat, turning them with tongs once, until they are bubbling and starting to blister, about 20 minutes. Remove from the oven and set aside to cool.
- Set the oven temperature at 350°F.
- Transfer the tomatoes and their juices from the baking sheet to a food processor fitted with a metal blade. Process in two or three quick pulses; the consistency should be chunky. Transfer to a bowl and set aside.
- In a large pot over high heat, bring 5 quarts water to a boil. In batches, add the red bell peppers and blanch for 1 minute or until just slightly softened. Remove with a spider or slotted spoon and set aside upside down in a colander to drain.
- In a large sauté pan or skillet over medium heat, warm the remaining 1/2 cup olive oil. Add the yellow and red onions and green bell peppers and sauté for 5 minutes, or until softened. Raise the heat to high and add the tempeh, cumin, red pepper flakes, and cayenne and sauté, stirring frequently, for 5 more minutes, or until the tempeh starts to brown. Add the roasted garlic and sauté for about 2 minutes. Remove from the heat and add the rice plus 2 cups of the processed tomatoes (reserve the rest for topping the finished peppers), the red wine vinegar, and thyme and stir well.
- Stuff the bell peppers with the rice mixture and transfer them to a baking dish into which they will fit snugly. Loosely cover with aluminum foil and bake for 30 minutes, or until the peppers are tender.
- Remove from the oven, evenly divide the remaining processed tomatoes by the number of peppers, and top the bell peppers with it. Garnish each pepper with a sprig of thyme and season with white pepper to taste.

GOOD GREEN TEMPEH PACKET

Yield: 2 servings

Soundtrack: "Surprise" by Kudu from *Kudu*

This dish can be made in advance and refrigerated for up to 2 days (it can also be frozen). Then, after a long day, you can pop one of these neat packets into your oven for 13 minutes and BAM! You're grubbin'.

1¼ cups packed flat-leaf parsley
  (1 cup chopped, ¼ cup minced)

4 cups 'Shroom Stock (page 79)

4 tablespoons extra-virgin olive oil

Coarse sea salt

½ pound tempeh
  (1 8-ounce package), cubed

½ bunch thick asparagus (about 8
  spears), trimmed and cut into 1-inch
  diagonals

1 cup packed minced spinach (a little less
  than 1 pound of spinach leaves)

½ cup white wine

Freshly ground white pepper

- In an upright blender, combine the parsley, 'Shroom Stock, 3 tablespoons olive oil, and 1 teaspoon salt and blend well for about 1 minute. Transfer to a medium-size saucepan and add the tempeh cubes. Over high heat, bring to a boil, immediately lower the heat to medium, and simmer for 1 hour, partially covered, until the tempeh is moist and saturated with broth. Remove from heat and drain in a colander.
- Preheat the oven to 375°F.

- Transfer the tempeh cubes to a parchment-lined baking sheet and roast for 20 minutes, stirring after 10 minutes for even browning.
- Raise the heat to 425°F.
- Bring 3 quarts of water to a boil in a large pot over high heat and add 1 teaspoon of salt. Add the asparagus and cook, uncovered, for 1 minute, until bright green.
- While the asparagus is boiling, prepare a large bowl of ice water to shock it.
- Remove the asparagus from the heat, drain, and immediately plunge into the ice water to stop the cooking. Drain and set aside.
- In a large bowl, combine the remaining olive oil, asparagus, the tempeh cubes, spinach, the remaining parsley, wine, and ¼ teaspoon salt. With clean hands, mix well for about 1 minute.
- Using wide aluminum foil, make a large packet by placing two sheets (a little larger than the size of a whole paper towel sheet) on top of each other, folding the bottom *up* and the two sides *in* a few times, and leaving the top open.
- Make sure that the mouth of the packet is wide open. With a serving spoon, transfer the contents of the bowl into the packet. Fold the top *over* a few times. Make sure that all the sides are folded tightly so everything can steam well.
- Place the packet on a baking sheet, transfer to a rack in the middle of the oven, and cook for about 13 minutes, until the vegetables are cooked.
- Remove from the oven. Transfer the packet to a platter, cut open with a knife, take a whiff, season with salt and pepper to taste, and serve with rice.

Seitan

WHOLE-GRAIN MUSTARD AND CORNMEAL CRUSTED SEITAN

Yield: 4 to 6 servings

Soundtrack: "Sound of Everything" by Quantic featuring Alice Russell from *Mishaps Happening*

Savory and crusty, this easy-to-prepare seitan dish makes for a tasty entrée along with a few sides. You can also dip the medallions in **Barbecue Sauce** (page 174) as an appetizer.

½ cup cornmeal

½ teaspoon fine sea salt

1 teaspoon freshly ground white pepper

¼ cup whole-grain mustard

1 pound (16 ounces) seitan, cut into ½-inch lengthwise medallions

½ cup extra-virgin olive oil

- Combine the cornmeal, salt, and pepper in a small bowl and whisk together with a fork. Set aside.

- Add the mustard to a small bowl. One at a time, using a pastry brush or your finger, rub the seitan medallions with mustard on all sides to lightly coat. Next dip the medallions in the cornmeal mixture, shaking off the excess cornmeal, and transfer to a clean plate.

- In a large sauté pan over medium-high heat, warm the olive oil. When the oil is hot but not smoking, add half of the seitan and fry until golden brown and crispy, 1 to 1½ minutes each side. Transfer to a paper towel–lined plate to drain. Repeat with the remaining medallions.

SMOTHERED SEITAN MEDALLIONS IN MIXED-MUSHROOM GRAVY

Yield: 4 to 6 servings
Soundtrack: "Brown" by Roy Hargrove from *Earfood*

I usually don't toot my own horn, but I have served this to a number of people who hold memories of smothered pork chops, and all of them have loved this dish. The seitan is succulent and the mushroom gravy is scrumptious.

- -

1 pound (16 ounces) seitan, cut into
  1/2-inch lengthwise medallions

5 tablespoons arrowroot powder

1 cup plus 2 tablespoons extra-virgin
  olive oil

1 large onion, sliced thinly

5 large cloves garlic, minced

2 cups **Mixed Mushroom Gravy**
  (page 181)

2 cups **'Shroom Stock** (page 79)

1 cup finely chopped green cabbage

2 jalapeños, seeded and minced

1/4 cup thinly sliced scallions

2 tablespoons minced parsley

- -

- Squeeze the seitan with a clean kitchen towel or paper towels to absorb excess moisture.
- Put the arrowroot powder in a small bowl.
- One at a time, dip the seitan pieces into the arrowroot powder, coating both sides. Shake off the excess and transfer the seitan to a large plate. Repeat until all the pieces are coated.
- In a large sauté pan over medium-high heat, warm 1/2 cup of the olive oil. When the oil is hot enough, add half of the seitan and fry until golden brown and crispy, 2½ to 3 minutes each side. Transfer to a paper towel–lined plate and drain. Drain the oil and its solids and discard. Add a fresh 1/2 cup of oil and repeat with the remaining seitan. Drain the oil and its solids and discard.
- Add the onions and the remaining olive oil to the sauté pan. Sauté over high heat, stirring often, until they cook down, 3 to 4 minutes. Immediately reduce the heat to medium and sauté gently, stirring occasionally, until soft, 8 to 10 minutes. Add the garlic and sauté until golden and fragrant, 2 to 3 minutes.
- Stir in the Mixed Mushroom Gravy and the 'Shroom Stock and bring to a boil. Immediately stir in the seitan and reduce the heat to medium low. Cover and simmer for 30 minutes.
- Add the cabbage, stir to incorporate, cover, and cook for 2 to 3 minutes. Stir in the jalapeño, scallions, and parsley. stir to incorporate, and cook for an additional minute.
- Remove from the heat and serve with rice.

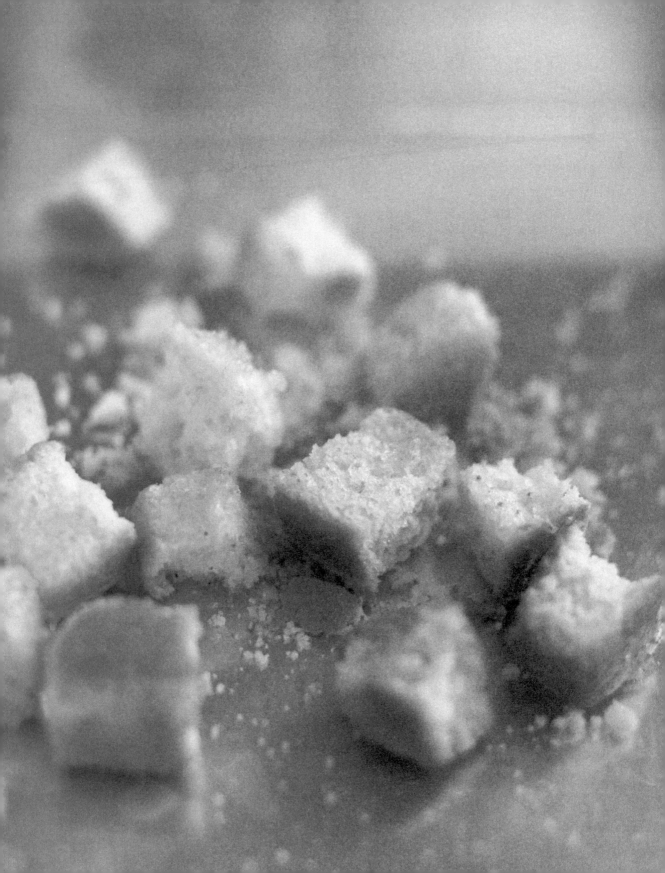

DAILY BREAD
BISCUITS. CAKES. CORNBREAD.

• Garlicky Cornbread Croutons •

• Johnny Blaze Cakes •

• Sweet Cornmeal-Coconut Butter Drop Biscuits •

• Quinoa-Quinoa Cornbread •

GARLICKY CORNBREAD CROUTONS

Soundtrack: "Southern Stuff" by Anthony Hamilton from *Ain't Nobody Worryin'*

In the spirit of recycling and reusing, I take leftover cornbread and make crunchy croutons that I add to soups and salads.

2 tablespoons extra-virgin olive oil

2 large cloves garlic, minced

2 large leftover pieces of **Quinoa-Quinoa Cornbread** (page 159) or your favorite cornbread cut into ½-inch cubes

- Preheat the oven to 350°F.
- In a medium-size sauté pan, combine the olive oil and the garlic. Turn the heat to medium-low and sauté for 3 to 5 minutes, until fragrant and golden. Remove from heat and set aside.
- In a large bowl, gently toss together the cornbread and the garlic oil. Transfer to a parchment-lined baking sheet and bake, shaking the pan a few times, until the croutons are golden brown, about 15 minutes. Set aside to cool.

JOHNNY BLAZE CAKES

Yield: 12 cakes
Soundtrack: "Bring the Pain" by Method Man from *Tical*

These crispy corn cakes are all-purpose. I sometimes serve them as an appetizer topped with **Rainbow Chow Chow** (page 182); as a main dish, I like them with **Chilled and Grilled Okra, Corn, and Heirloom Tomato Salad** (page 68) heaped on top; and of course you can't go wrong serving these with **Strawberry and Slightly Hot Pepper Jam** (page 177) for breakfast.

1½ cups stone-ground cornmeal
½ cup whole wheat pastry flour
1 teaspoon baking powder
1 teaspoon fine sea salt
¼ teaspoon cayenne
2½ cups boiling unflavored rice milk
2 jalapeños, seeded and minced
Extra-virgin olive oil

- In a large bowl, combine the cornmeal, flour, baking powder, salt, and cayenne. Set aside.
- In a small saucepan, bring the rice milk to a boil then slowly pour it over the cornmeal mixture, stirring as you pour. Add the jalapeño to the batter, mix well, and refrigerate the batter for 20 minutes.
- Preheat the oven to 250°F.
- Warm a large, nonstick skillet or a griddle over medium-high heat and grease well with 1 tablespoon of olive oil. Add ¼ cup of batter to the skillet per cake. A large skillet should comfortably fit two to three. After about 1 minute, when the bottom starts to set, reduce the heat to medium-low, and use a wooden spoon to shape the cakes, pushing them in and up so that they are about 3 inches wide and ½ inch thick. Cook the cakes for 8 to 10 minutes per side, adding more oil after turning, until they are golden brown and crispy on the outside (do this in several batches). Transfer the cooked cakes from the skillet to a baking sheet and keep them warm in the oven until all the cakes are cooked.

SWEET CORNMEAL-COCONUT BUTTER DROP BISCUITS

Yield: about 24 biscuits
Soundtrack: "Turn Left" by Little Dragon from *Little Dragon*

3/4 cup whole wheat pastry flour

3/4 cup unbleached white flour

1/2 cup medium grind cornmeal

2 tablespoons organic raw cane sugar

2 teaspoons baking powder

1/2 teaspoon baking soda

1/2 teaspoon ground cinnamon

1/2 teaspoon fine sea salt

6 tablespoons chilled coconut butter

3/4 cup original unflavored rice milk

2 tablespoons pure maple syrup

1 tablespoon apple cider vinegar

- Preheat the oven to 425°F.

- In a large bowl, sift together the flours, cornmeal, sugar, baking powder, baking soda, cinnamon, and salt. Rub the coconut butter into the flour mixture with your fingertips until the mixture resembles sand with pebbles.

- Combine the rice milk, maple syrup, and apple cider vinegar and mix well. Then, make a well in the center of the flour pebbles, add the rice milk, and stir just until the dough comes away from the sides of the bowl.

- Drop walnut-sized balls of dough from a spoon onto a parchment-lined baking sheet and bake for 10 to 12 minutes, or until lightly browned.

QUINOA-QUINOA CORNBREAD

Yield: 4 to 6 servings
Soundtrack: "Se Me Van Los Pies" by Susana Baca from *Susana Baca*

Inspired by Myra Kornfeld's "Amaranth-Studded Cornbread" from her brilliant book *The Voluptuous Vegan*, this recipe uses quinoa flour as well as whole quinoa, which gives it a rich, nutty flavor and some crunch. You can find them both at health food supermarkets. Up until now quinoa didn't show up often in African American–inspired cuisine, but this is a new day. . . .

- -

5 tablespoons unrefined corn oil,
  plus more for oiling the pan

1/4 cup quinoa

3/4 cup cornmeal

1/2 cup quinoa flour

1/2 cup unbleached all-purpose flour

1 teaspoon baking powder

1 teaspoon baking soda

1/2 teaspoon salt

1 cup original unflavored rice milk

2 tablespoons apple cider vinegar

1/4 cup agave nectar

- -

- Set a rack in the middle of the oven and preheat to 425°F.
- Grease an 8-inch-square bread pan and set aside.
- In a medium-size skillet over medium heat, toast the quinoa, shaking the pan occasionally, until the grains start to pop, 2½ to 3 minutes. Transfer the quinoa to a large bowl.
- Add the cornmeal, quinoa flour, all-purpose flour, baking powder, baking soda, and salt to the bowl with the toasted quinoa. Whisk to combine.
- In a separate bowl, whisk together the rice milk, apple cider vinegar, agave nectar, and 5 tablespoons of corn oil.
- Transfer the bread pan to the oven to preheat until sizzling, about 5 minutes.
- After the pan has heated for 4 minutes, combine the wet mixture with the dry mixture with a large spoon and quickly mix just until the dry ingredients are moist. Do not overmix or the bread will be dense.
- Remove the pan from the oven and immediately scrape the batter into it. Return the pan to the oven and bake on the center rack for 15 to 18 minutes, or until the cornbread is golden brown and firm to the touch (and a toothpick inserted into the middle comes out cleanly).
- Serve immediately.

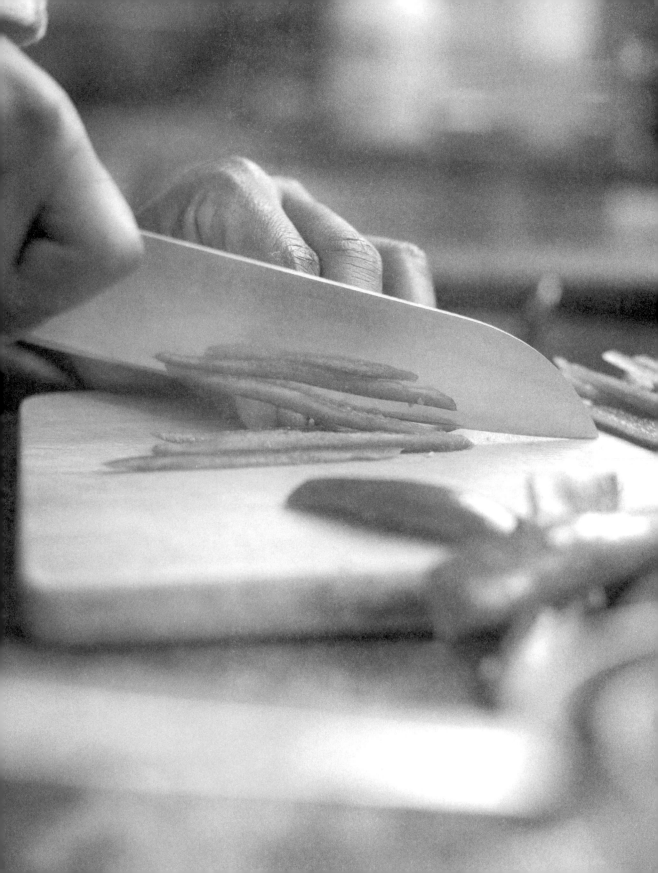

MARGIE'S CUPBOARD
CONDIMENTS. SAUCES. PRESERVES. PICKLES.

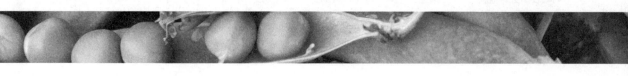

- Herbed Sea Salt -
- Cajun-Creole Spice Blend -
- Hot Apple Cider Vinegar -
- Garlic Olive Oil -
- Multipurpose Coating for Dredging Foods -
- Creamed Cashews -
- Mixed-Herb Marinade -
- Creamy Celeriac Sauce -
- Hot Pepper Sauce -
- Basic Tomato Sauce -
- Fresh Plum Ketchup -
- Barbecue Sauce -
- Caramelized Red Onion Relish -
- Peach Salsa -
- Strawberry and Slightly Hot Pepper Jam -
- Spicy Dill Pickles -
- Smoky Pickled Purple Okra -
- Green Tomato–Basil Chutney -
- Mixed Mushroom Gravy -
- Rainbow Chow Chow -

HERBED SEA SALT

Yield: about ¼ cup
Soundtrack: "Sprinkle Me" by E-40 and Suga T from *In a Major Way*

The first time I had herbed salt was when Nigel Walker of Eatwell Farm gave me some of his lavender salt. After that, I started experimenting with other herbs, even combining some to make mixed herb sea salts. My favorite is basil sea salt, which I make to sprinkle on **Watermelon Slices with Basil Sea Salt** (page 16). If your salt starts to cake up, simply give it another whirl in the grinder.

2 tablespoons finely chopped fresh herbs of your choice
¼ cup coarse sea salt

- In a coffee grinder, combine the herbs and salt. Pulse until mixed well. Store in an airtight glass container.

CAJUN-CREOLE SPICE BLEND

Yield: about 1/2 cup

Soundtrack: "Cissy Strut" by The Meters from *The Meters*

1 tablespoon onion powder

5 teaspoons garlic powder

1 tablespoon paprika

1 tablespoon chili powder

2 teaspoons red pepper flakes

1/2 teaspoon cayenne

1 tablespoon dried thyme

1 tablespoon dried oregano

1 tablespoon coarse sea salt

1 tablespoon black peppercorns

- Combine all the ingredients in a spice grinder and grind to a powder.
- Store in a tightly sealed jar.

A QUICK GUIDE TO CANNING/PRESERVING FOOD

At first glance, canning seems to be a daunting task, but it's actually pretty simple and fun. Once you get into the groove of it you will be flexing your canning muscles all summer so you will have plenty of food to put away for leaner winter months. Here are a few tips to get you started.

The right jars

You will need to get some special canning jars that you can usually buy in bulk (they are the ones with the lids and rings that come apart when you open them). My favorite brand is Kerr and I sometimes use Ball.

Keep it clean and hot

It is essential to sterilize your jars before storing any food in them (whether you plan to seal the jars or not) along with any utensils that you will be using during processing. The best way to do this is by simmering your jars, lids, rings, and utensils in boiling water. You can purchase special canning tongs (with a rubber grip) to handle hot items. After I boil everything, I remove them to a clean baking sheet and hold them in an oven set at the lowest temperature possible.

We need to process

Once you have loaded your jars up with tasty treats you can store them in the refrigerator or you can process them in a bath of hot water to seal the jar. Once sealed, store them in a dark cabinet, pantry, or similar cool, dark storage space. Always keep food stored in the refrigerator unless the recipe states that it can be stored in a pantry. Preserved items have to include the right amount of sugar and salt in order for them to preserve properly and not spoil.

To process: Set a metal rack at the bottom of a large stockpot. Fill the pot with water and bring to a boil. Using canning tongs, carefully transfer enough filled jars to the rack to fit comfortably, ensuring that the jars are covered by about 2 inches of water. Cover and boil for the amount of time called for in the recipe. Carefully transfer the jars from the pot to a work surface until they cool to room temperature and the lids seal (they should be concave). Store sealed containers in a cool, dark cabinet or cupboard for up to one year. Refrigerate any jars that do not seal properly and enjoy.

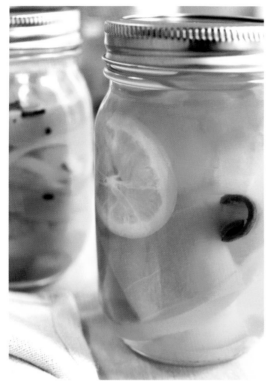

Citrus and Spice Pickled Watermelon Rind • page 20

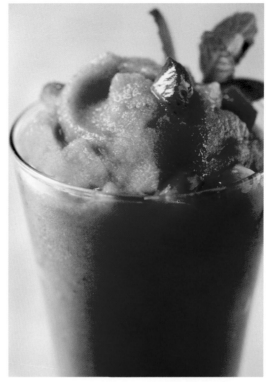

Double Watermelon–Strawberry Slushee • page 18

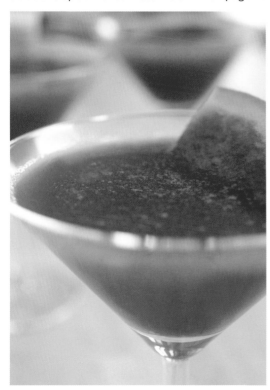

Fresh Watermelon–Vodka Martini • page 17

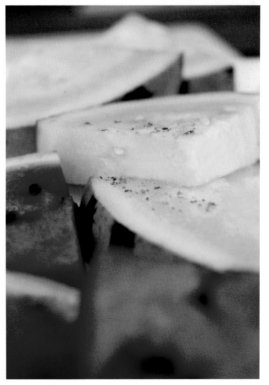

Watermelon Slices with Basil Sea Salt • page 16

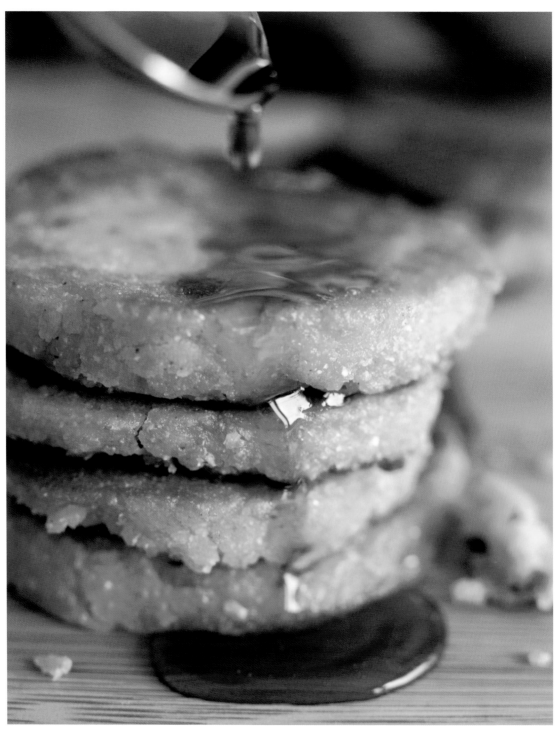

Johnny Blaze Cakes • page 157

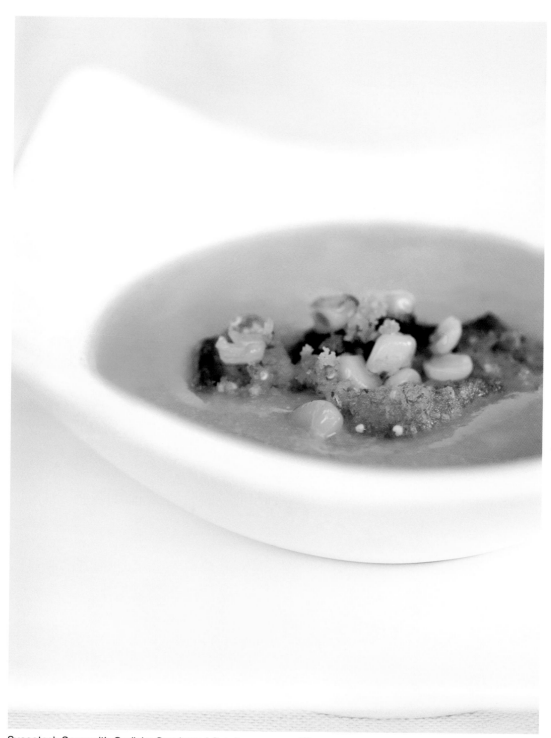

Succotash Soup with Garlicky Cornbread Croutons • page 88

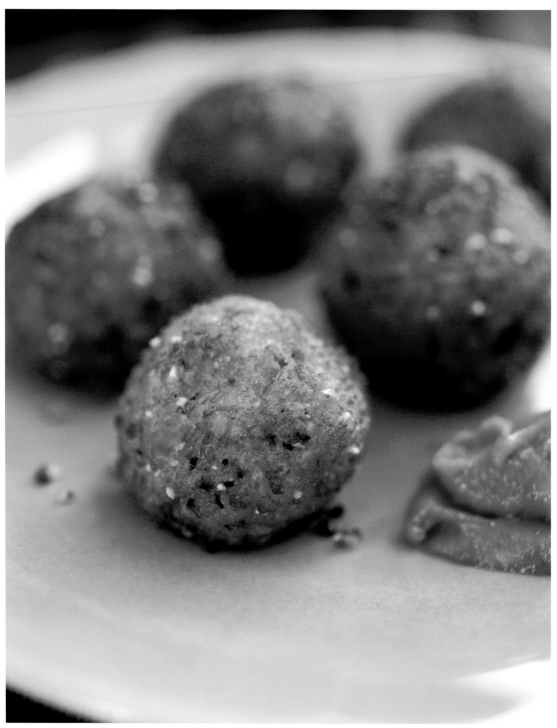

Black-Eyed Pea Fritters with Hot Pepper Sauce • page 48

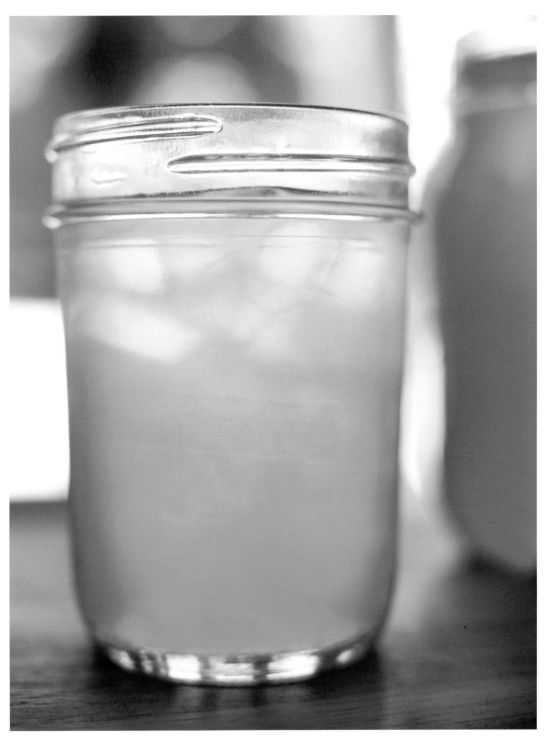

Agave-Sweetened Orange-Orange Pekoe Tea • page 5

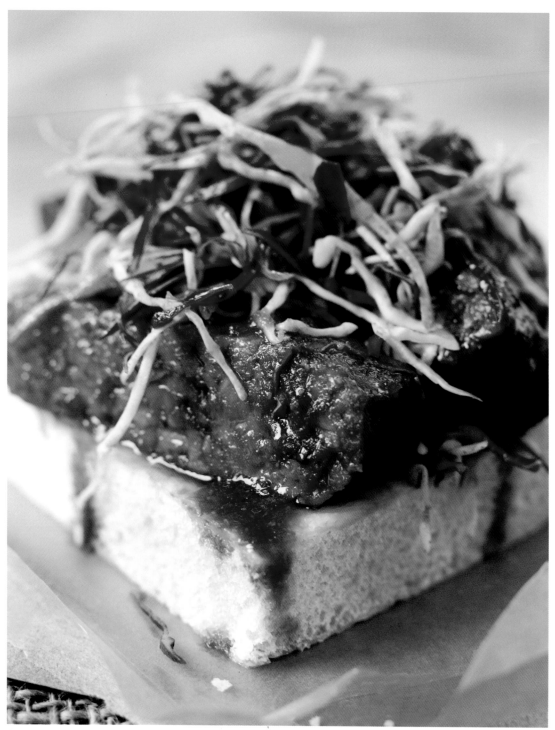

Open-Faced BBQ Tempeh Sandwich with Carrot-Cayenne Coleslaw • page 12

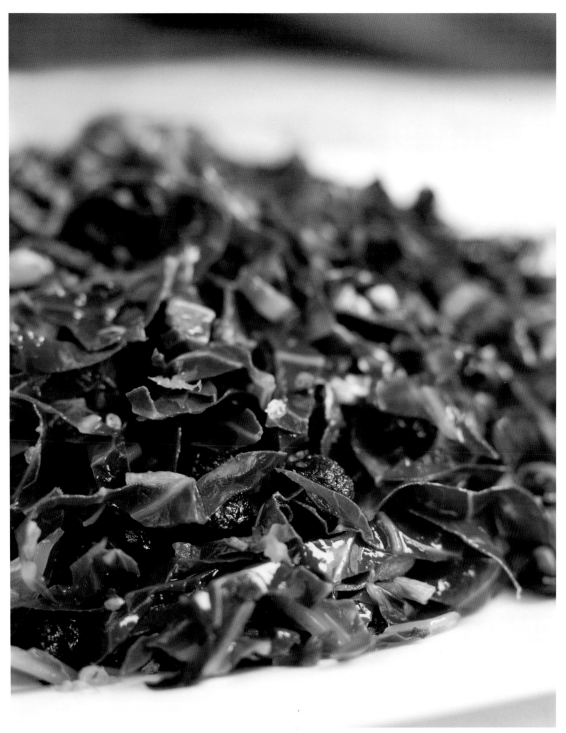

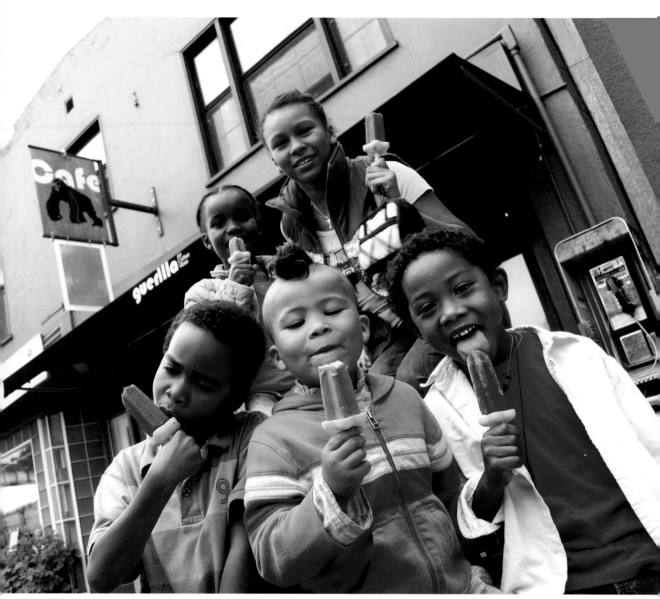

Soul on Ice Pops • page 186

HOT APPLE CIDER VINEGAR

Yield: about 1 pint
Soundtrack: "Game Is My Middle
Name" by Betty Davis from *Betty Davis*

My family keeps a bottle of "hot vinegar"
on hand so that we can add a few dashes to
greens right before eating.

2 cups of apple cider vinegar

1 dried chipotle chile, sliced thinly

- Add enough apple cider vinegar to reach
  the neck of a sterilized, pint-size canning
  jar. Add the chile (seeds and all). Cover
  tightly.
- Store in a cool, dark pantry for seven days,
  seven hours, and seven minutes, agitating
  at least once per day.

GARLIC OLIVE OIL

Yield: 1 cup
Soundtrack: "Who Rize Above" by Dragons of Zynth from *Coronation Thieves*

This can be used whenever olive oil is called for to infuse a dish with garlic flavor.

1 cup extra-virgin olive oil
10 large cloves garlic, chopped finely

- In a small saucepan, combine the oil and the garlic. Turn the heat to the lowest point at which the oil will simmer and cook for 30 minutes.
- Strain the oil into a sterilized canning jar and let cool.
- Store in the refrigerator for up to one month.

MULTIPURPOSE COATING FOR DREDGING FOODS

Yield: 2 cups

Soundtrack: "Fried Neck Bones and Some Homefries" by Willie Bobo from *Verve Unmixed 2*

I use this coating for dredging **Crispy Okra Strips with Lime-Thyme Vinaigrette** (page 46) and **Fried Green Tomatoes with Creamy Celeriac Sauce** (page 110).

½ cup whole wheat pastry flour

1 cup cornmeal

1 teaspoon fine sea salt

2 teaspoons freshly ground white pepper

¼ teaspoon cayenne

- In a large resealable plastic bag, combine the flour, cornmeal, salt, pepper, and cayenne. Shake well to blend.
- That's it.
- Be sure to store any remaining coating in the freezer, as it will go rancid otherwise.

CREAMED CASHEWS

Yield: 1 cup

Soundtrack: "Cariño (Chico Mann Remix)" by Ocote Soul Sounds / Adrian Quesada from *The Alchemist Manifesto**

Although native to Brazil, the majority of cashews sold in America come from India and East Africa. Soaking these sweet-tasting nuts for a few hours and then pureeing them with water in an upright blender renders a smooth blend that I use as a dairy-free substitute for heavy cream to give dishes a creamy consistency and more depth. I also use it in fruit smoothies to add protein and make them creamier. Look for whole cashews that are white and crisp.

1 cup cashews, soaked overnight and drained

½ cup water

- In an upright blender, combine the cashews and water and blend until smooth.

MIXED-HERB MARINADE

Yield: about 3¼ cups
Soundtrack: "Africian Herbsman" by Bob Marley & The Wailers from *African Herbsman*

This simple, fresh marinade is an excellent match with **Mixed-Herb-Marinated Grilled Summer Squash and Bell Peppers** (page 105) or tofu when grilling. After using, the marinade can be frozen and used at a later date.

¼ cup freshly squeezed lemon juice

¾ cup freshly squeezed orange juice

¾ cup freshly squeezed lime juice

½ cup apple juice

2 tablespoons minced fresh basil

2 tablespoons minced fresh parsley

2 tablespoons minced fresh rosemary

2 cloves garlic, minced

2 serrano chiles, seeded and minced

1½ teaspoons coarse sea salt

½ cup olive oil

- In a large bowl, combine all the ingredients and whisk well.

CREAMY CELERIAC SAUCE

Yield: about 2 cups
Soundtrack: "Three Changes" by
The Good, The Bad & The Queen from
The Good, The Bad & The Queen

Inspired by rémoulade, a condiment often served with seafood dishes, I created this sauce for the dishes **Fried Green Tomatoes with Creamy Celeriac Sauce** (page 110) and **Pan-Fried Coconut-Tempeh Cubes with Creamy Celeriac Sauce** (page 50), but it also goes nicely with **Grilled Asparagus with Rosemary Sea Salt** (page 103). This will keep up to three days refrigerated.

½ pound silken tofu
¼ cup freshly squeezed lemon juice
1 tablespoon minced parsley
1 clove garlic, minced
½ teaspoon agave nectar
½ teaspoon Dijon mustard
2 tablespoons extra-virgin olive oil
1 teaspoon paprika
⅛ teaspoon cayenne
Coarse sea salt
Freshly ground white pepper
¼ cup minced scallions
½ cup peeled and coarsely grated
   celery root (celeriac)

- In an upright blender, combine the tofu, lemon juice, parsley, garlic, agave nectar, mustard, olive oil, paprika, cayenne, ½ teaspoon salt, and ¼ teaspoon white pepper and blend until smooth. If necessary, season with additional salt and pepper to taste.
- Transfer the sauce to a bowl and stir in the scallions and celery root.

HOT PEPPER SAUCE

Yield: 1 cup
Soundtrack: "Hot Lava" by Kudu from *Death of the Party*

This is my attempt to replicate the oh-so-slammin' hot sauce at the Senegalese restaurant Joloff, my favorite eatery in New York City. This version is only slightly hot, but if you really want that fire add one more habanero chile.

¼ cup extra-virgin olive oil

1 small red onion, diced

½ teaspoon cumin

⅛ teaspoon cayenne

Coarse sea salt

1 large clove garlic, minced

1 habanero chile, minced

¼ cup tomato paste

¼ cup tomato sauce

2 teaspoons apple cider vinegar

¼ cup water

¼ teaspoon freshly ground
   white pepper

- In a saucepan over low heat, warm the oil. Add the onion, cumin, cayenne, and ½ teaspoon salt and sauté until the onions start to caramelize, about 8 minutes.

- Stir in the garlic and chile and sauté for 2 minutes more. Add the tomato paste, tomato sauce, vinegar, and water. Mix well, and simmer until it starts to thicken, about 5 to 7 minutes.

- Transfer all the ingredients to an upright blender, add the white pepper, and puree until smooth. Season with additional salt to taste. Store in a tightly sealed jar in the refrigerator.

BASIC TOMATO SAUCE

Yield: about 3 cups
Soundtrack: "Pressure" by Killer Mike featuring Ice Cube from *I Pledge Allegiance to the Grind II*

While I'm an advocate of using fresh vegetables as much as possible, I'm fine with using canned tomatoes for making sauces and adding to dishes. I use this as a topping for my **Rosemary-Roasted Tofu Cubes** (page 146) and as a base for pizzas.

3 tablespoons extra-virgin olive oil
1 teaspoon oregano
1/4 teaspoon red pepper flakes
1/2 teaspoon coarse sea salt
2 large cloves garlic, minced
1 28-ounce can diced tomatoes
1/2 teaspoon balsamic vinegar

- In a medium-size saucepan, combine the olive oil, oregano, red pepper flakes, salt, and garlic. Turn the heat to medium-high and sauté for 1 minute, stirring frequently.
- Stir in the tomatoes, raise the heat, and bring to a boil. After 30 seconds reduce the heat to medium-low and simmer for 15 minutes, stirring every few minutes. Add the balsamic vinegar, cook for an additional minute, and remove from heat. If necessary, add additional salt.

FRESH PLUM KETCHUP

Yield: about 2½ cups
Soundtrack: "Percolator" by Stereolab from *Emperor Tomato Ketchup*

This sweet ketchup is a tastier version of store-bought ketchup without all the additives and preservatives.

1 tablespoon extra-virgin olive oil

½ cup diced red onion

½ cup diced red bell pepper

¼ teaspoon paprika

2 cloves garlic, minced

1 8-ounce can chopped tomatoes

½ teaspoon agave nectar

1 tablespoon red wine vinegar

2 teaspoons tamari

3 ripe plums, peeled, pit removed, and chopped

3 tablespoons freshly squeezed lemon juice

Coarse sea salt

Freshly ground white pepper

- In a large sauté pan over medium heat, combine the olive oil, onion, bell pepper, and paprika. Sauté for 8 to 10 minutes, stirring often, until the vegetables begin to caramelize. Add the garlic and sauté until fragrant, about 2 minutes. Add the tomatoes, agave, vinegar, and tamari. Reduce the heat to low, cover, and simmer, stirring occasionally, until thickening, about 15 minutes. Remove from the heat. Stir in the plums and lemon juice and set aside to cool.
- Transfer the ketchup to an upright blender and puree until smooth. Season with salt and pepper to taste.
- Store in an airtight container in the refrigerator for up to a week.

BARBECUE SAUCE

Yield: about 2 cups

Soundtrack: "The Frim Fram Sauce" by Ella Fitzgerald and Louis Armstrong from *Ella & Friends*

This sauce goes really well with aussen fay and chafafa on the side, and I enjoy it wherever I would use barbecue sauce.

¼ cup extra-virgin olive oil

¼ cup red wine vinegar

¼ cup freshly squeezed lime juice

¼ cup tamari

1 8-ounce can tomato sauce

2 large chipotle chiles, canned in adobo sauce

¼ cup agave nectar

1 tablespoon ground cumin

⅛ teaspoon cayenne

1 teaspoon dried thyme

½ cup water

- Combine all the ingredients in an upright blender and puree for 30 seconds.
- In a saucepan over medium-high heat, simmer the sauce, stirring often, until it has reduced and thickened to 2 cups.
- Store in the refrigerator in an airtight container.

CARAMELIZED RED ONION RELISH

Yield: 2 cups
Soundtrack: "Cry Me a River" by Dinah Washington (Truth and Soul Remix) from *Verve Remixed, Vol. 4*

I made this sweet, tasty relish to go with **Mixed-Herb-Marinated Grilled Summer Squash and Bell Peppers** (page 105), but you can use it wherever you would enjoy a relish.

1 tablespoon extra-virgin olive oil

4 cups sliced red onions

¼ teaspoon coarse sea salt

2 teaspoons agave nectar

2 tablespoons apple cider vinegar

2 tablespoons water

Freshly ground white pepper

- In a small skillet over low heat, combine the oil, the onions, and salt and sauté, stirring often, until the onions are well caramelized, about 30 minutes.
- Stir in the remaining ingredients and bring to a boil. Reduce heat and simmer, uncovered, for 10 minutes, stirring often.
- Transfer to a bowl, cover, and refrigerate until cool.

PEACH SALSA

Yield: 3 cups
Soundtrack: "My Favorite Things" by Sarah Vaughan from *After Hours*

I think it's a shame not to take advantage of fresh peaches when they are in season, so I try to create as many dishes as possible using them. This salsa can be enjoyed wherever you would use a tomato salsa.

1 small red onion, diced

2 cups diced peaches

3 tablespoons minced fresh cilantro

1 jalapeño, seeded and minced

2 tablespoons freshly squeezed orange juice

2 tablespoons freshly squeezed lime juice

½ teaspoon coarse sea salt

- In a large bowl, combine all the ingredients, toss well, and refrigerate, covered, for 30 minutes to allow flavors to marry.
- Serve immediately.

STRAWBERRY AND SLIGHTLY HOT PEPPER JAM

Yield: about 1 pint
Soundtrack: "Peter Piper" by Run-DMC from *Raising Hell*

In addition to sweetening jams, sugar acts as a preservative. So most jams contain too much sugar for my taste. Here, I reduce the amount of sugar and use apple cider as an additional sweetener. Using less sugar in this jam means that it won't last as long as one traditionally prepared. So refrigerate it and use it within two weeks (but I doubt that it will last that long). In terms of fruit, a good rule of thumb is this: only use strawberries that you would thoroughly enjoy eaten by themselves. So purchasing ripe strawberries when they are in season will be your best bet. You won't get enough of **Johnny Blaze Cakes** (page 157) topped with this.

---

1 tablespoon freshly squeezed lemon juice

1 tablespoon apple cider vinegar

1 habanero chile, seeded and minced

2 tablespoons arrowroot powder

3/4 cup plus 3 tablespoons apple cider

2 cups organic raw cane sugar

1 pound medium organic strawberries, washed, dried, hulled, and halved

---

- In a medium-size saucepan, combine the lemon juice, vinegar, and the chile. Turn the heat to medium and simmer, reducing the mixture until about 1 tablespoon remains, about 1 1/2 minutes. Remove from the heat and set aside.

- In a small bowl, combine the arrowroot powder with 3 tablespoons of apple cider and mix well until the arrowroot powder is dissolved. Transfer to the saucepan with the lemon-vinegar-chile mixture and add the remaining apple cider, the sugar, and the strawberries.

- Turn the heat to low and cook the mixture, stirring frequently with a wooden spoon, until all the sugar has dissolved, about 5 minutes. Next, raise the heat to medium-low and simmer, without stirring, for 15 minutes. Remove from the heat and stir a few times. Cool completely.

- Ladle into a sterilized pint-size canning jar (page 164) and refrigerate.

SPICY DILL PICKLES

Yield: 6 pints

Soundtrack: "Dill Pickle Tango" by The Microscopic Septet from *Surrealistic Swing—History of the Micros, Vol. 2*

1 cup coarse sea salt

1½ gallons plus 3 cups water

18 Kirby cucumbers (no more than 4 inches long), quartered lengthwise

3 tablespoons red pepper flakes

1 tablespoon yellow mustard seeds

1 tablespoon cumin seeds

1 tablespoon coarsely ground white pepper

3 cloves garlic, minced

½ cup apple cider vinegar

3½ cups distilled white vinegar

2 tablespoons agave nectar

2 bunches dill, minced

- In a large stockpot over medium-low heat, make a brine by combining 3/4 cup of the salt with 1½ gallons of water. Stir well until the salt is completely dissolved. Remove from heat and set aside to cool. Add the cucumbers to the brine, place a small plate on top to ensure that they are completely covered in the water, and refrigerate overnight.

- Drain the cucumbers in a colander, rinse with cold water, and set aside.

- In a small sauté pan over medium heat, combine the red pepper flakes, mustard seeds, cumin seeds, and pepper and toast until fragrant, about 2 minutes. Transfer to a large saucepan. Stir in the garlic, vinegars, agave nectar, dill, and the remaining salt and water. Simmer until the salt is dissolved, about 3 minutes. Set aside to cool.

- Divide the cucumbers evenly between the sterilized canning jars (page 164).

- Leaving ½ inch of space at the top, fill the jars with the vinegar mixture. Close the jars with the lids and rings. Store jars in a refrigerator for at least forty-eight hours before eating.

SMOKY PICKLED PURPLE OKRA

Yield: 6 pints
Soundtrack: "African Student Movement" by Saul Williams from *Saul Williams*

----

3 pounds young, small-to-medium purple okra pods (green will work, but purple is prettier), stems cut off

6 tablespoons kosher salt

6 cloves garlic, whole

1½ teaspoons whole peppercorns

3½ cups white distilled vinegar

½ cup apple cider vinegar

2 cups water

4 large dried chipotle chiles, ground into powder

- Wash the okra.

- In a large pot, bring 4 quarts of water to a boil, add 2 teaspoons salt, and boil the okra for 2 minutes. Drain.

- Place 1 clove garlic and ¼ teaspoon of peppercorns in the bottom of each sterilized canning jar (page 164).

- Divide the blanched okra evenly among the six canning jars and stuff them tightly inside (placing some stems up and others down will allow you to fit more inside).

- In a medium-size saucepan over medium heat, bring the vinegars, water, chile powder, and the remaining salt to a boil. Immediately remove the mixture from the heat and pour it over the okra in the jars, leaving ½ inch of space at the top.

- Close the jars with the lids and rings.

- Process in a hot bath for 10 minutes (page 164).

- Store in a cool, dark, and dry place for at least two weeks before enjoying.

GREEN TOMATO–BASIL CHUTNEY

Yield: 3 cups

Soundtrack: "Beloved" by Anoushka Shankar (Thievery Corporation Remix) from *Rise Remixes* EP

Light and tangy, this chutney makes a tasty supplement to any meal.

2 tablespoons extra-virgin olive oil

2 cloves garlic, minced

2 teaspoons ground cumin

1/2 habanero chile, seeded and minced

4 cups green tomatoes, cut into 1/2-inch dice (about 6 tomatoes)

2 teaspoons agave nectar

Coarse sea salt

1 tablespoon red wine vinegar

1 tablespoon minced basil

Freshly ground white pepper

- In a medium-size saucepan, combine the olive oil, garlic, cumin, and chile. Turn the heat to medium-low and gently sauté, stirring often, until the garlic is fragrant and golden, about 3 minutes.
- Add the tomatoes, raise the heat to high, and bring to a boil. Immediately reduce the heat to low and simmer until the liquid starts to thicken, about 15 minutes.
- Add the agave, 1/2 teaspoon sea salt, the vinegar, and the basil and simmer, stirring occasionally, for 1 minute.
- Season with salt and white pepper to taste.

MIXED-MUSHROOM GRAVY

Yield: 2 cups
Soundtrack: "Groovy Gravy" by Quincy Jones from *The Original Jam Sessions 1969*

Although created for the **Smothered Seitan Medallions in Mixed-Mushroom Gravy** (page 153), I also pair it with simple mashed potatoes, plain brown rice, and other gravy-worthy dishes.

2 tablespoons extra-virgin olive oil

1/4 pound button mushrooms

1/4 pound baby bella mushrooms

2 tablespoons whole wheat pastry flour

1 cup unflavored rice milk

1 cup **'Shroom Stock** (page 79)

Coarse sea salt

Freshly ground white pepper

- In a medium-size saucepan over medium-low heat, warm 1 tablespoon of the oil, add the mushrooms, and sauté for 5 minutes, stirring often. Add the flour and the remaining olive oil and stir until well combined. Reduce the heat to low and cook, stirring often, until the flour starts to brown, about 10 minutes.
- While whisking, add the rice milk, the 'Shroom Stock, 1/2 teaspoon salt, and 1/2 teaspoon white pepper. Simmer until thickened, whisking constantly, about 15 minutes.
- Season with additional salt and pepper to taste.

RAINBOW CHOW CHOW

Yield: 6 pints (3 quarts)
Soundtrack: "Rainbow Country" by
Bob Marley & The Wailers from *The
Complete Upsetter Collection—Bob Marley
& The Wailers*

Ma'Dear's not-to-be-forgotten Chow
Chow consisted of cabbage, peppers, green
tomatoes, and finely chopped onions that
was cooked for five hours and served with
leafy greens such as collards, mustards, or
turnips. This colorful condiment is not
slow-cooked like hers, but it is equally
tasty eaten with beans, greens, and other
vegetables.

1 cup apple cider vinegar

1 cup white distilled vinegar

1 cup water

2½ cups organic raw cane sugar

¼ cup coarse sea salt

1 tablespoon yellow mustard seeds

3 tablespoons dry mustard

1 teaspoon celery seed

1 teaspoon turmeric

1½ pounds green cabbage

1½ pounds red cabbage

1 pound green bell peppers, seeded and
cut into ¼-inch dice

1 pound orange bell peppers, seeded
and cut into ¼-inch dice

1 pound red bell peppers, seeded and
cut into ¼-inch dice

1 pound yellow bell peppers, seeded and
cut into ¼-inch dice

4 jalapeños, seeded and cut into
¼-inch dice

1½ pounds green tomatoes, cut into
¼-inch dice

2 pounds yellow onions, cut into
¼-inch dice

- In a large saucepan, bring the vinegars, water, sugar, salt, mustard seeds, dry mustard, celery seeds, and turmeric to a boil. Reduce heat to medium and simmer for 30 minutes, stirring occasionally.
- Add the cabbage, bell peppers, jalapeño, green tomatoes, and onions to the saucepan. Bring back to a boil, immediately reduce the heat to medium low, and simmer until the relish starts to thicken, about 25 minutes.
- Spoon the relish into the six pint-size canning jars, leaving 1/2 inch of space at the top.
- Close the jars with the lids and rings.
- Process in a hot bath for 25 minutes (page 164).

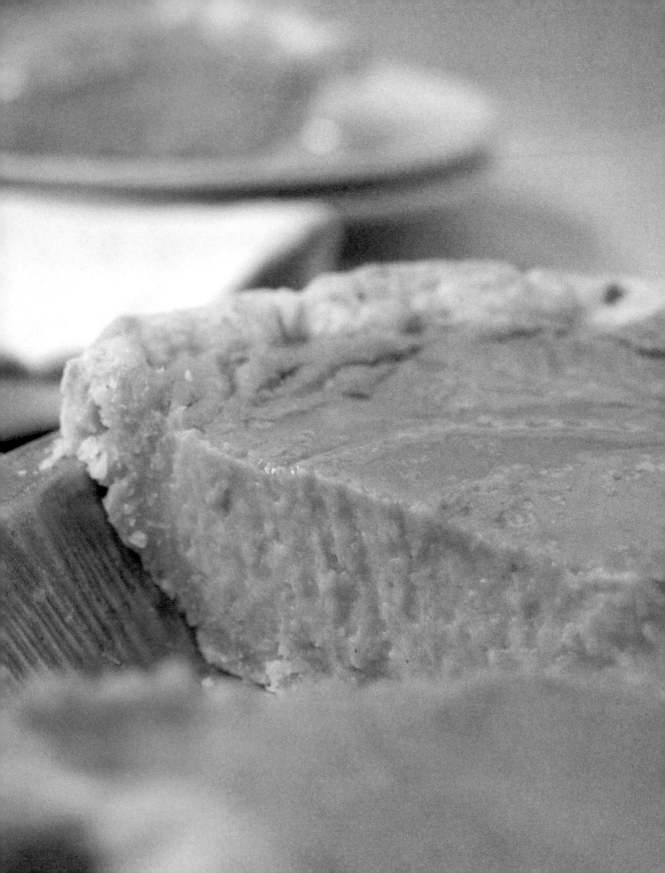

SWEET THANGS
DESERTS. CANDIES. AMBROSIAL TREATS.

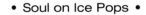

• Soul on Ice Pops •

• Coconut Oil Pie Crust •

• Balsamic Peaches with Creamed Cashews •

• Candied Orange Peel •

• Chocolate-Orange Pudding •

• Chocolate-Pecan Pudding Pie •

• Chocolate-Granola Pudding Parfait •

• Coconut-Pecan Pralines •

• Maple Yam-Ginger Pie •

• Molasses-Vanilla Ice Cream with Candied Walnuts •

• Spiced Peach Rustic Pie with Dried Cranberries •

SOUL ON ICE POPS

Soundtrack: "I Can" by Nas from *God's Son* and "Soul on Ice" by Me'Shell Ndegeocello from *Plantation Lullabies*
Book: *Soul on Ice* by Eldridge Cleaver (Delta, 1999)

My grown-up popsicle kick started when I bought molds online from Williams-Sonoma to freeze **Chocolate-Orange Pudding** (page 190) and make Chocolate-Orange Pudding Pops. I then started experimenting with different beverages to see what worked best. My favorites so far are made from **Sin-ger [sin jer] Thirst-Quencher** (page 34) and fresh watermelon juice (page 16). I learned the hard way that there is a distinction between kids and grown-up Soul on Ice Pops. Kids generally have a preference for lemonade-based pops and chocolate pudding pops (they aren't feeling ginger that much).

When making yours, pour fresh juice or drink into the mold, leaving ¼ inch space at the top to allow for expansion after freezing, and place the pops in a freezer for at least 6 hours, until frozen completely. When I make them for kids I usually add a little agave nectar or **Simple Syrup** (page 26) before freezing, as I find that freezing beverages decreases their sweetness. Your call.

COCONUT OIL PIE CRUST

Yield: 1 crust

Soundtrack: "I Want You" by Erykah Badu from *Worldwide Underground*

This is an all-purpose crust that can be used for desserts as well as savory dishes like potpies. I use this one for the **Maple Yam-Ginger Pie** (page 194). This crust will last for two days refrigerated and up to two weeks in the freezer.

1/2 cup whole wheat pastry flour

1/2 cup unbleached all-purpose flour

1/2 teaspoon baking powder

2 teaspoons raw organic cane sugar

1/4 teaspoon fine sea salt

7 tablespoons coconut butter (solidified coconut oil)

1 teaspoon apple cider vinegar

1/4 cup ice water

- Combine the flours, baking powder, sugar, and salt in a bowl. Whisk to combine. Add the solid coconut oil into the bowl and rub it into the flour mixture with your fingers until the mixture resembles small pebbles.

- Add the cider vinegar to the ice water. Drizzle the water into the dough 1 tablespoon at a time, mixing in each as you add it. You should stop adding water when the dough holds together when squeezed, and make sure not to add any more water than necessary.

- Transfer to a clean surface. Shape the dough into a ball and then flatten into a disc. Wrap in plastic wrap and refrigerate for 45 minutes.

BALSAMIC PEACHES WITH CREAMED CASHEWS

Yield: 4 servings
Soundtrack: "Microphone Fiend" by Eric B. & Rakim from *Follow the Leader*

Simmering fresh peaches in the balsamic-orange marinade and serving them with a dollop of **Creamed Cashews** (page 168) puts this dish halfway between breakfast and dessert. I'll let you decide.

4 fresh peaches, halved and pitted

1/2 cup balsamic vinegar

1/2 cup freshly squeezed orange juice

2 tablespoons agave nectar

Creamed Cashews (page 168)

- Place all the peaches cut side down in a large casserole dish.
- In a medium-size bowl, combine the balsamic vinegar, orange juice, and agave nectar. Mix well.
- Pour the marinade over the peaches and let them absorb it for 15 minutes.
- In a large sauté pan over high heat, add the peaches, cut side down, along with the marinade and cook for 3 minutes, until softened.
- Remove the peaches to a plate.
- Over high heat, continue cooking the marinade, stirring occasionally, until it reduces to a syrup, 3 to 5 minutes.
- For each serving, transfer two peach halves to a plate, add a dollop of Creamed Cashews, and drizzle some of the syrup over and around the peaches.

CANDIED ORANGE PEEL

Yield: about 4 cups
Soundtrack: "Gimme" by Jill Scott from *Experience—Jill Scott 826+*

Don't throw away those orange peels (or other citrus peels). Save them to make this tasty snack both kids and adults can't get enough of. As you can imagine, they are really sweet. But I occasionally have one or two as an after-dinner treat. Most often, though, I use them to sweeten my **Cinnamon-Applejack Toddy** (page 35) and other hot teas. I also add them to ice cream and sorbets when I really want to be bad.

---

4 whole orange peels or other citrus peels (the thicker the better), washed, and cut into quarters

1¾ cups organic raw cane sugar

1 cup water

- In a medium-size saucepan over medium-high heat, combine the peels with enough water to cover them by 2 inches and bring to a simmer for 1 hour, until tender.
- Drain and rinse under cold water until cool. With the edge of a spoon, scrape away any remaining pulp or pith. Cut the peels into as many strips as possible that are 2 inches long and ¼ inch wide (others can be shorter and oddly shaped). Set aside.
- In a medium-size saucepan over low heat, combine ¾ cup of the sugar and 1 cup of water and bring to a simmer, stirring frequently with a wooden spoon, until the sugar is completely dissolved.
- Add the peels and simmer until most of the syrup has been absorbed, about 1 hour.
- Transfer the peels to a sieve or a colander and drain.
- Spread the remaining sugar over a large plate. Roll each peel in the sugar individually and then transfer to parchment paper to dry for 6 hours or overnight.

CHOCOLATE-ORANGE PUDDING

Yield: 4 to 6 servings
Soundtrack: "Addiction" by Kanye West from *Late Registration*

I have a lot of friends rearing dairy-free kids, so I created this version of one of my childhood favorites (minus the unwholesome ingredients found in most commercial puddings) to share with them. Psych! I created it for myself.

6 tablespoons coconut milk

½ cup agave nectar

½ teaspoon orange extract

½ cup unsweetened cocoa powder

⅛ teaspoon fine sea salt

2 boxes (¾ pound) Mori-Nu firm silken tofu (this dessert only works with this brand because of its particular texture)

- In a medium-size saucepan, combine the coconut milk, agave nectar, orange extract, cocoa powder, and salt and whisk to incorporate the cocoa powder. Bring to a boil over high heat and then immediately reduce the heat to low and simmer for 1 minute, whisking constantly. Remove from the heat.

- Pour the mixture into in a blender, add the tofu, and blend until smooth. Transfer to a medium bowl.

- Cover with plastic and refrigerate for 1 hour to cool down.

CHOCOLATE-PECAN PUDDING PIE

Yield: 8 servings
Soundtrack: "Pillz" by Jaylib from *Champion Sound*

Coming home from Memphis a few years ago, I stumbled on an immediately mouth-watering recipe for Chocolate Pecan Pie (in of all places the airport!). The recipe had all the usual unhealthy trappings of Southern food: lots of "bad" fat and highly processed sugars. But by the time I got home, I had figured out which health-supportive ingredients could be substituted for the less healthy ones. I decided to use maple syrup, for instance, instead of light corn syrup. In the end, the only resemblance that my pie had with the original one was chocolate and pecans.

3/4 cup unflavored rice milk

1/4 cup arrowroot powder

1/2 banana

3/4 cup nondairy chocolate chips

1/2 cup pure maple syrup

1 teaspoon vanilla extract

1/4 cup coconut oil

1 1/4 cups pecans, chopped

1/2 cup dried unsweetened coconut

1 **Coconut Oil Pie Crust** (page 187)

Mint leaves, for garnish

- In a blender, combine the rice milk and arrowroot powder and puree for 30 seconds. Add the banana and puree for 15 seconds. Set aside.
- In the top of a double boiler over simmering water, melt the chocolate chips. In a large bowl, immediately combine the melted chocolate chips with the rice milk mixture, maple syrup, vanilla extract, coconut oil, pecans, and dried coconut. Mix well and set aside.
- Preheat the oven to 425°F.
- Unwrap the pie dough and transfer it to a lightly floured surface. With a rolling pin, roll the dough into a 12-inch circle. Roll the dough onto the pin and unroll it into a 9-inch pie plate. Gently press the dough into the bottom and sides of the plate. Trim the edges with a knife. Make a decorative edge on the crust by pressing a piece of the dough between the forefinger of one hand and the thumb and forefinger of the other. Repeat this continuously around the edge of the entire pie.
- Wrap the edge of the crust with aluminum foil to prevent it from burning and prick the bottom of the crust with a fork several times. Transfer the crust to the oven and prebake for 5 minutes.
- Remove the crust from the oven, scrape the filling into it with a rubber spatula, and spread evenly.
- Place the pie on a cookie sheet and bake for 20 minutes, until filling is firm.
- Remove from the oven, cool for 30 minutes, then refrigerate for at least two hours.
- Garnish each slice with a few mint leaves.

CHOCOLATE-GRANOLA PUDDING PARFAIT

Yield: 2 servings
Soundtrack: "Love Is Blindness" by Cassandra Wilson from *New Moon Daughter*

Chocolate-Orange Pudding (page 190)

Maple-Almond Granola (page 129)

- Place two parfait or comparable glasses in the freezer for 1 hour.
- In each glass, place 3 tablespoons of Chocolate-Orange Pudding at the bottom. Top with 3 tablespoons of Maple-Almond Granola. Repeat until you have three layers of each (six layers total) in each glass.
- Refrigerate until ready to enjoy.

COCONUT-PECAN PRALINES

Yield: about 9 pralines
Soundtrack: "Red House" by
Jimi Hendrix from *Blues*

Along with coffee and beignets from Café
Du Monde in New Orleans, pralines (pro-
nounced [PRAH-leens] or [PRAW-leens] or
[PRAY-leens]) were one of my weaknesses
during college days. No matter how you
pronounce it, this sugar-filled dessert is
decadent and delicious. Since they are
mostly sugar, I only break these out on special occasions like Mardi Gras, so as not to
tempt myself too often.

1 cup pecan halves

1½ cups organic raw cane sugar

½ cup coconut milk

¼ teaspoon vanilla extract

1 teaspoon coconut butter

2 tablespoons dried unsweetened
coconut

⅛ teaspoon fine sea salt

- Preheat the oven to 375°F.
- Spread the pecans on a large baking
  sheet and toast for 6 minutes, stirring
  halfway through the cooking.
- In a medium-size saucepan over high
  heat, combine the sugar and coconut milk
  and bring to a boil while stirring constantly
  with a wooden spoon.
- When the temperature reaches 228°F on a
  candy thermometer, stir in the vanilla extract, coconut butter, dried coconut, salt,
  and pecans and continue to cook, stirring
  constantly, until the mixture reaches 236°F.
- Remove the pan from the heat and cool
  for 5 minutes.
- Beat the mixture with a wooden spoon until the candy coats the pecans but does
  not lose its gloss.
- To make the pralines, drop the mixture
  2 tablespoons at a time onto parchment
  paper. Allow the pralines to fully cool until
  completely solid, about 1 hour.
- Enjoy responsibly.

MAPLE YAM-GINGER PIE

Yield: 8 to 10 servings (4 to 6 greedy)
Soundtrack: "Cold Turkey" by Anthony David from *Acey Duecy*

Instead of replicating the classic sweet potato pie, I use yams. I only add a touch of ginger, as not to overshadow the main ingredient.

---

1 **Coconut Oil Pie Crust** (page 187)

2½ pounds garnet yams, peeled

2 cups coconut milk

1 tablespoon plus 2 teaspoons agar flakes

2 teaspoons minced fresh ginger

¼ cup plus 2 tablespoons pure maple syrup

1 teaspoon vanilla extract

1 teaspoon ground cinnamon

½ teaspoon freshly grated nutmeg

2 tablespoons arrowroot powder

½ teaspoon fine sea salt

- Remove the pie crust dough from the re-frigerator and allow it to warm to room temperature.
- In a large pot over high heat, combine the yams with cold water to cover by a few inches. Bring to a rolling boil and cook until the yams can be easily pierced with a fork, about 40 minutes. Remove from heat and drain. Measure out 2 cups of the cooked yams and set aside (reserve the rest of the yams and eat them as a side dish.)

- In the meantime, unwrap the pie dough and transfer it to a lightly floured surface. With a rolling pin, roll the dough into a 12-inch circle. Roll the dough onto the pin and unroll it into the pie plate. Gently press the dough into the bottom and sides of the plate. Trim the edges with a knife. Make a decorative edge on the crust by pressing a piece of the dough between the fore-finger of one hand and the thumb and forefinger of the other. Repeat this contin-uously around the edge of the entire pie.
- Preheat the oven to 400°F.
- Wrap the edge of the crust with aluminum foil to prevent it from burning and prick the bottom of the crust with a fork several times. Transfer the crust to the oven and pre-bake for 6 to 8 minutes, until golden brown. Remove and set aside.
- Lower the temperature of the oven to 375°F.
- In a saucepan over medium heat bring the coconut milk to a simmer (do not let boil). Add the agar flakes and the ginger and simmer for 8 minutes, stirring often, until the agar dissolves. Stir in the maple syrup and vanilla extract and simmer for an addi-tional minute. Turn off the heat.
- Add the yams, agar mixture, cinnamon, nutmeg, arrowroot, and the fine sea salt to a food processor fitted with a metal blade. Process until creamy and smooth.
- Pour the filling into the pie shell and smooth the top with a wet spatula. Bake for 25 to 30 minutes, until the filling is firm.
- Cool on a wire rack for 2 hours, or until the pie has firmed up.

MOLASSES-VANILLA ICE CREAM WITH CANDIED WALNUTS

Yield: 3$1/2$ cups
Soundtrack: "Sweet Thing" by Chaka Khan & Rufus from *Rufus Featuring Chaka Khan*

Because dark molasses is high in calcium, iron, and potassium, I occasionally make lemonade using it as a sweetener, but the drink is more medicinal than anything else. The distinctive and often overpowering flavor of molasses tends to be too strong and not to my liking. But I wanted to use molasses in at least one dessert, since my grandmother used to sweeten cakes and pies with it back in the day. So I tested this recipe a few times using molasses as a sweetener and found the right balance to give this ice cream a subtle caramel flavor.

3 cups coconut milk

2 tablespoons arrowroot powder

6 tablespoons agave nectar

1 tablespoon dark molasses

2 teaspoons vanilla extract

$1/8$ teaspoon fine sea salt

1 cup **Candied Walnuts** (page 40), chopped

- In a small cup, mix $1/4$ cup of the coconut milk with the arrowroot powder to make a slurry. In a medium-size saucepan over medium heat, combine the remaining coconut milk, agave nectar, molasses, vanilla extract, and salt with the coconut milk slurry. Warm until starting to thicken, 2 to 3 minutes.

- Transfer to the refrigerator until completely cold.

- Pour into an ice cream maker and freeze creamy, 25 to 30 minutes. Add the walnuts for the last minute of freezing. Transfer to an airtight container and place in freezer until firm, about 2 hours.

SPICED PEACH RUSTIC PIE WITH DRIED CRANBERRIES

Yield: 6 to 8 servings
Soundtrack: "Be Healthy" by Dead Prez from *Let's Get Free*

This flavorful cobbler deserves only the freshest and ripest peaches, so please avoid using canned ones. You can, however, substitute fresh nectarines.

Filling

3½ pounds ripe peaches, peeled, pitted, and cut into ½-inch dice

½ cup cold apple juice

2 tablespoons plus 1 teaspoon arrowroot powder

1 teaspoon cinnamon

½ teaspoon freshly grated nutmeg

2 teaspoons freshly squeezed lemon juice

¼ cup plus 2 tablespoons agave nectar

1 teaspoon lemon zest

½ cup dried cranberries

⅛ teaspoon fine sea salt

Crust

1¾ cups unbleached all-purpose flour, chilled

¾ cup whole wheat pastry flour, chilled

3 tablespoons organic raw cane sugar

½ teaspoon fine salt

½ teaspoon baking powder

½ cup plus 3 tablespoons coconut butter

½ cup plus 2 tablespoons ice water

For the filling

- Place the peaches in a large bowl. In a small bowl, combine 3 tablespoons of the apple juice with the arrowroot powder, cinnamon, and nutmeg and mix well until the arrowroot powder and spices are thoroughly blended. Transfer to the bowl with the peaches. Add the lemon juice, agave nectar, lemon zest, cranberries, salt, and the remaining apple juice and toss well with clean hands.
- Transfer the peach mixture to a large saucepan. Over medium heat, cook the mixture, stirring constantly, until it begins to thicken, about 10 minutes. Remove from the heat and set aside to cool.

For the pastry

- Combine the flours, sugar, salt, and baking powder in a large bowl and mix well. Add the coconut butter to the flour mixture and rub with your fingertips until the mixture resembles fine sand.
- Drizzle the water into the dough 1 tablespoon at a time, mixing in each as you add it. You should stop adding water when the dough holds together when squeezed and make sure not to add any more water than necessary.
- Divide the dough in half, squeeze each half into a tight ball, and flatten each half into the shape of a square. Wrap each square in plastic and let rest in the refrigerator for at least 45 minutes.

- Preheat the oven to 375°F.
- Remove one of the dough squares from the refrigerator and roll it out on a lightly floured work surface until it is about 2½ inches larger than a 2-quart (2-inch-deep) baking dish on all sides and about 1/8 inch thick. Transfer the dough to the baking dish, covering the bottom and fitting the dough up the sides. Poke a few holes in the dough on the bottom of the baking dish with a fork. Trim off the excess dough and tear it into small pieces. Transfer them to a parchment-lined baking sheet.
- Transfer the baking sheet and the baking dish to the oven. Bake until the pieces (about 15 minutes) are golden brown and the crust (about 25 minutes) is browning.
- Add the baked pieces to the peach mixture and stir to combine. Transfer the mixture to the baked crust.
- Remove the second dough square from the refrigerator and roll it out on a lightly floured work surface until it is about 1/2 inch larger than the baking dish. Drape the dough over the top surface and neatly tuck it inside the baking dish. Make seven small slits in the pastry crust to allow steam to escape.
- Bake the cobbler on the middle oven rack for 1 hour, or until the crust is crisp and golden brown and the fruit filling is bubbling. Transfer the cobbler to a wire rack and let it cool for at least 1 hour.

BIG UPS

To the one, my angels, and my ancestors (upon your shoulders I stand) for your guidance.

To my parents, Beatrice and Booker Terry, and my sister Jamelah Terry, M.D. (proud of you Jay Jay), for your unwavering belief in and support of me. Always. You're my foundation.

To all my extended family members—the Bryants and the Terrys. Major props to Uncle Don for writing the prayer-song to open this book.

To my brilliant, beautiful, and 'bout it-'bout it fiancée, Jidan Koon, for showing me that the revolution is LOVE. We are doing it big—and for forever!!!!!

To Marilyn Wong and Wang-Sang Koon for all of your love and support.

To Danfeng, Jando, and Chencho for leading by example.

To all the extended Wong family for your support.

To the late Edna Lewis, Peter Berley, Anne-marie Colbin, Jessica B. Harris, Jamie Oliver, Melvin Van Peebles, and Alice Waters for inspiration.

To all my teachers and mentors for your wisdom and guidance.

To my literary agent Danielle Svetcov for believing in me and this project from day one, providing expert editing, and giving sagacious advice on many fronts.

To Jim Levine, Arielle Eckstut, Monika Verma, and the whole Levine-Greenberg team for your hard work and support.

To my editor Renée Sedliar for seeing and supporting my vision from our first hour-long conversation in the summer of 2007 'til now and for constantly pointing me in the right direction. I look forward to makin' BIG THANGS happen.

To John Radziewicz, Matthew Lore, and the whole team at Da Capo/Perseus for your support and for publishing bomb-ass books.

To Myra Kornfeld for offering to support this project based upon a paragraph description.

To Yanna Flemming for creating my fly Web sites, helping me "manage my brand identity," and being a down friend.

To the amazingly brilliant Sara Remington for always being up for going on an adventure and making beautiful art. We're takin' over, sun.

To Keba Konte for taking a beautiful photograph of the youth.

To the youths: Assata, Fela, Indigo, M'kai, and Mbire for being down for the cause (and thanks to their parents).

To Rebecca Stevens and Lori Camille for kitchen assistance.

To my kick-butt assistant Shayna Marmar for all your hard work (thank you, thank you, thank you, thank you, thank you, thank you, thank you so much).

To my accountant Joe Cornwall for going above and beyond duty.

To my colleagues at the Food and Society Policy Fellows Program for your inspiration and support.

To the Fair Food Foundation and Oran Hesterman for financial support.

To AEPOCH and Laura Loescher for financial support and friendship.

To Peter Barnes and The Common Counsel Foundation for providing a beautiful space for writers to retreat.

To Youth for Environmental Sanity (YES!) and the Robbins family for all the support you have shown me over the years.

To Bioneers and Arty Mangan for your support.

To the staff and faculty at the Natural Gourmet Institute for Health and the Culinary Arts for your support.

To Lynette Clemetson, Terry Samuel, and the rest of the team at theroot.com for giving me a platform.

To Bruce Cole and Bonnie Powell at *Edible San Francisco* for your support (thanks for the cover!).

To Added Value, People's Grocery, Farm Fresh Choice, Oakland Food Connection, the Food Project, Growing Power, Community Services Unlimited, RIC, and all the food justice organizations holdin' it down across the nation.

To Anna Lappé for always dreaming big with me.

To Mike Molina for always pushing me to be great.

To Michelle Rhone-Collins, Joseph Collins, Marla Teyolia, and Will Power for supporting me from the beginning.

To my sisters Ludie Minaya, Elizabeth Johnson, and Latham Thomas for being on my team.

To Ferentz Lafargue for always being down for reading my essays and offering suggestions for improvements.

To my fellow Mesa Refuge writers, Linda Faillace and Josh Kun for your feedback, great advice, and company.

To Curt Kurzenhauser for providing me with a ridiculously beautiful home in San Francisco to rest, write, and test recipes for seven months.

To Savannah Shange and Greg Cluster for opening up "the house" to me in the summer of 2007 and beyond.

To all my folks in Memphis, New Orleans, New York, the Bay Area, Los Angeles, Santa Fe, Atlanta, Baltimore, and everywhere in between for your support.

Allen, Patricia. *Together at the Table: Sustainability and Sustenance in the American Agrifood System.* University Park: Pennsylvania State University Press, 2004.

Berley, Peter. *Fresh Food Fast.* New York: Regan Books, 2004.

———. *The Modern Vegetarian Kitchen.* New York: Regan Books, 2004.

Colbin, Annemarie. *Food and Healing.* New York: Ballantine Books, 1986.

Edge, John T. *The New Encyclopedia of Southern Culture, Vol. 7: Foodways.* Chapel Hill: University of North Carolina Press, 2007.

Harris, Jessica B. *The Welcome Table: African-American Heritage Cooking.* New York: Simon & Schuster, 1996.

Katz, Sandor Ellix. *The Revolution Will Not Be Microwaved: Inside America's Undergrounds Food Movements.* White River Junction, VT: Chelsea Green Publishing, 2006.

Kingsolver, Barbara, Camille Kingsolver, and Steven L. Hopp. *Animal, Vegetable, Miracle: A Year in the Life of Food.* New York: HarperCollins, 2007.

Kornfeld, Myra. *The Voluptuous Vegan: More Than 200 Sinfully Delicious Recipes for Meatless, Eggless, and Dairy-Free Meals.* New York: Clarkson Potter, 2004.

Lappé, Anna, and Bryant Terry. *Grub: Ideas for an Urban Organic Kitchen.* New York: Tarcher, 2006.

Lewis, Edna. *The Taste of Country Cooking: 30th Anniversary Edition.* New York: Knopf, 2006.

Moskowitz, Isa Chandra, and Terry Hope Romero. *Veganomicon: The Ultimate Vegan Cookbook.* New York: Da Capo Press, 2007.

Nestle, Marion. *Food Politics: How the Food Industry Influences Nutrition and Health.* Berkeley: University of California Press, 2007.

———. *What to Eat.* New York: North Point Press, 2007.

Oliver, Jamie. *Cook with Jamie.* New York: Hyperion, 2008.

Opie, Frederick Douglass. *Hog and Hominy: Soul Food from Africa to America.* New York: Columbia University Press, 2008.

Pollan, Michael. *In Defense of Food: An Eater's Manifesto.* New York: Penguin, 2008.

Reid, Daniel P. *The Tao of Health, Sex, and Longevity: A Modern Practical Guide to the Ancient Way.* New York: Fireside, 1989.

Robbins, John. *Healthy at 100: The Scientifically Proven Secrets of the World's Healthiest and Longest-Lived Peoples.* New York: Ballantine Books, 2007.

Schatz, Halé Sofia, and Shira Shaiman. *If the Buddha Came to Dinner: How to Nourish Your Body to Awaken Your Spirit.* New York: Hyperion, 2004.

Shiva, Vandana. *Stolen Harvest: The Hijacking of the Global Food Supply.* Cambridge, MA: South End Press, 2000.

Swanson, Heidi. *Supernatural Cooking: Five Ways to Incorporate Whole and Natural Ingredients into Your Cooking.* Berkeley: Celestial Arts, 2007.

Waters, Alice. *The Art of Simple Food: Notes, Lessons, and Recipes from a Delicious Revolution.* New York: Clarkson Potter, 2007.

Williams-Forson, Psyche A. *Building Houses Out of Chicken Legs: Black Women, Food, and Power.* Chapel Hill: University of North Carolina Press, 2006.

Wood, Rebecca. *The New Whole Foods Encyclopedia: A Comprehensive Resource for Healthy Eating.* New York: Penguin, 1999.

_____

INDEX

ABOUT THE AUTHOR

Bryant Terry is an eco chef, food justice activist, and author. For the past eight years he has worked to build a more just and sustainable food system and has used cooking as a tool to illuminate the intersections between poverty, structural racism, and food insecurity. His interest in cooking, farming, and community health can be traced back to his childhood in Memphis, Tennessee, where his grandparents inspired him to grow, prepare, and appreciate good food.

Bryant is currently a fellow of the Food and Society Policy Fellows Program, a national project of the W. K. Kellogg Foundation and the Fair Food Foundation. He has garnered many honors and awards for his work including receiving the inaugural Natural Gourmet Institute Award for Excellence in Health-Supportive Food Education and being selected as one of the 2008 "Hot 20 under 40" in the San Francisco Bay Area by *7x7 magazine*. Bryant's first book (coauthored with Anna Lappé), *Grub: Ideas for an Urban Organic Kitchen,* won a 2007 Nautilus Award for Social Change.

Bryant contributes essays and recipes to a number of online and print outlets, and his work has been featured in *Gourmet, Food and Wine,* the *New York Times Magazine,* the *San Francisco Chronicle, Vibe, Domino,* and many other publications. Bryant has a regular column—"Eco-Soul Kitchen"—on theroot.com. He has made dozens of national radio and television appearances (Fox, NBC, PBS, BET, and Sundance), including making a guest appearance on the eco-reality series *Mario's Green House* and being a host on "The Endless Feast," a thirteen-episode series that explores the connection between the earth and the food on our plates.

In 2001, Bryant founded b-healthy! (Build Healthy Eating and Lifestyles to Help Youth), a four-year initiative designed to empower youth to be active in creating a more just and sustainable food system. Along with Ludie Minaya, Elizabeth Johnson, and Latham Thomas, Bryant helped illuminate the importance of cooking as a tool for organizing and base building for the food justice movement.

Bryant completed the Chef's Training Program at the Natural Gourmet Institute for Health and Culinary Arts in New York City. He holds an M.A. in American History from New York University and a B.A. with honors in English from Xavier University of Louisiana.

He lives and creates in Oakland with his brilliant, beautiful, and 'bout it-'bout it fiancée, Jidan Koon, and their bird, Kiwi.

www.bryant-terry.com

———

CONTRIBUTORS

Best known as a staff songwriter at Hi Records and as the husband of Hi Records star Ann Peebles, **Don Bryant** was born in Memphis on April 4, 1942; his father, Edward, sang with a gospel group called the Four Stars of Harmony, and Bryant himself began singing in church at age five. At Hi Records, Bryant co-wrote a number of Peebles's signature songs, including "I Can't Stand the Rain" and "99 Pounds," and he penned material for other Hi Records stars including Al Green, Syl Johnson, O. V. Wright, and Otis Clay. In 1986 Bryant released a gospel album, *What Do You Think about Jesus?*, and in 2000, he recorded another gospel album, *It's All in the Word.*

www.myspace.com/donbryant

Myra Kornfeld is the author of *The Healthy Hedonist Holidays: A Year of Multi-Cultural Vegetarian-Friendly Holiday Feasts*, *The Voluptuous Vegan*, and *The Healthy Hedonist*. Kornfeld has written for *Natural Health* magazine and *Organic Style* and is a frequent contributor to *Vegetarian Times*. She teaches classes in ethnic, classic, and vegetarian cooking at the *Natural Gourmet School of Food and Health and the Institute of Culinary Education* in New York City. A veteran restaurant chef and consultant, Kornfeld worked for six years creating innovative vegan cuisine at New York's Angelica Kitchen. Kornfeld specializes in cooking parties and team-building events and is currently the "taster, tester and tweaker" for a food and health Web site called **myfoodmyhealth.com**.

San Francisco-born **Keba Konte** is an Oakland-based artist and co-owner of Guerilla Café—an art café in the Gourmet Ghetto of North Berkeley, California. He received degrees in Photojournalism and Black Studies from San Francisco State University and in Digital Photography from the San Francisco Multimedia Studies Program. He has exhibited his work in numerous solo and group shows throughout California and the United States. Konte and his work have been featured in the *Los*

Angeles Times, San Francisco Chronicle, Up-scale, Colorlines, SFSU, Code, Oprah at Home, Oakland Tribune, and *Oakland Magazine,* as well as a myriad of journals and books including the *International Review of African American Art, Reflections in Black: A History of Black Photographers, 1840 to the Present, Hands,* by Bernard Dadie, and *Nueva Luz Photographic Journal.* Accolades include the 2006 Alameda County Art Commission Public Art Mural Award, Jack London Square Public Art Awards, SOHO PHOTO Alternative Processes Competition Exhibition Award, the En Foco New Works Photography Award, and the prestigious commission to create the artwork for the 2003 Amnesty International/Sierra Club "Defending the Defenders" poster campaign to raise awareness of the human rights of international environmentalists.

www.kebakonte.com

Michael Otieno Molina is an author, educator, performer, publisher, and mixed-media artist born and raised in New Orleans. With degrees in English from Xavier Univesity of Louisiana and law from Yale Law School, Michael is founder of Second Line Publishing and the New Roots New Orleans youth writing program, as well as writer, producer, and actor in a short film adaptation of writings from his blog and novella, *Purgatory Stories* (www.purgatorystories.blogspot.com).

Michael is a nationally recognized performer, public speaker, and author of books *The Second Line; Water Meter: A Glossary of New Orleans Terms to Know;* and *The Good Favor Social Aid and Pleasure Club.*

www.momolina.org

Sara Remington was raised in upstate New York and moved to California after years of being trapped in piles of snow. With inspiration derived from the beauty of raw, unprocessed foods, organic ingredients, natural light, and fresh air, Sara has the "ability to tell stories with such poignantly simple, yet elegant images that speak volumes" (*Digital Photo Pro*). She was honored by Photo District News as one of the "30 Emerging Photographers of 2006" and continues to shoot for editorial, advertising, and book publishing firms worldwide. Sara is based in the San Francisco Bay Area.

She is currently working on a book about the Big Sur Bakery for HarperCollins, and she also has an ongoing personal project titled "Swordfish," photographing hundreds of nostalgic objects from her grandparents' house in upstate New York. When she is not shooting, you can find Sara driving up and down the coast on Highway 1, climbing rocks all over California, and enjoying anchovies and a really stinky cheese.

www.sararemington.net

Brittany Moira Powell was born in Naples, Italy. Since then, she has lived in many parts of the country, including New Orleans and the Washington, D.C., area, thanks to her military father and her accommodating mother. After graduating from the California College of Arts and Crafts (now CCA), with a degree in photography, she settled in Oakland, CA. Brittany loves surfing, and photographing the people closest to her, and she has recently expanded her subject matter to include strangers and the great outdoors.

www.brittanympowell.com

———

DIGESTIF
EAT. THINK. ACT.

As parents, educators, advocates, and people who just care, we have to understand that the best place to recruit soldiers for what Alice Waters calls the "Delicious Revolution" is at the dinner table. That's why for the past eight years, my overriding approach to the issues of health, food, and farming has been: *Start with the visceral, move to the intellectual, and end with the political.*

More than giving talks, facilitating workshops, or writing articles or a book, I found that I moved the most people to shift their relationship with food by making them a delicious meal using grub (healthy, local, sustainably raised food for all). Sure, just before we dig in, I might mention the health benefits of eating foods in season, or the economic consequences of supporting small farmers, or the environmental impact of eating locally. But after that, I sit back and let people get their grub on. Inevitably, the questions about those issues roll in.

Consumer action is important, and if we want to impact the food system as a whole, we have to call upon our elected officials to create policies that will ensure that our children and grandchildren inherit a food supply that is more secure, diverse, and healthy than the one we now have. As citizens, we vote with our ballots; as consumers, we vote with our forks. For more information and ideas visit the "Learn and Act" section on www.eatgrub.org.

METRIC CONVERSIONS

- The recipes in this book have not been tested with metric measurements, so some variations might occur.
- Remember that the weight of dry ingredients varies according to the volume or density factor: 1 cup of flour weighs far less than 1 cup of sugar, and 1 tablespoon doesn't necessarily hold 3 teaspoons.

General Formulas for Metric Conversion

Ounces to grams	⇒ ounces × 28.35 = grams
Grams to ounces	⇒ grams × 0.035 = ounces
Pounds to grams	⇒ pounds × 453.5 = grams
Pounds to kilograms	⇒ pounds × 0.45 = kilograms
Cups to liters	⇒ cups × 0.24 = liters
Fahrenheit to Celsius	⇒ (°F − 32) × 5 ÷ 9 = °C
Celsius to Fahrenheit	⇒ (°C × 9) ÷ 5 + 32 = °F

Linear Measurements

½ inch = 1½ cm
1 inch = 2½ cm
6 inches = 15 cm
8 inches = 20 cm
10 inches = 25 cm
12 inches = 30 cm
20 inches = 50 cm

Volume (Dry) Measurements

¼ teaspoon = 1 milliliter
½ teaspoon = 2 milliliters
¾ teaspoon = 4 milliliters
1 teaspoon = 5 milliliters
1 tablespoon = 15 milliliters
¼ cup = 59 milliliters
⅓ cup = 79 milliliters
½ cup = 118 milliliters
⅔ cup = 158 milliliters
¾ cup = 177 milliliters
1 cup = 225 milliliters
4 cups or 1 quart = 1 liter
½ gallon = 2 liters
1 gallon = 4 liters

Volume (Liquid) Measurements

1 teaspoon = ⅙ fluid ounce = 5 milliliters
1 tablespoon = ½ fluid ounce = 15 milliliters
2 tablespoons = 1 fluid ounce = 30 milliliters
¼ cup = 2 fluid ounces = 60 milliliters
⅓ cup = 2⅔ fluid ounces = 79 milliliters
½ cup = 4 fluid ounces = 118 milliliters
1 cup or ½ pint = 8 fluid ounces = 250 milliliters
2 cups or 1 pint = 16 fluid ounces = 500 milliliters
4 cups or 1 quart = 32 fluid ounces = 1,000 milliliters
1 gallon = 4 liters

Oven Temperature Equivalents, Fahrenheit (F) and Celsius (C)

100°F = 38°C
200°F = 95°C
250°F = 120°C
300°F = 150°C
350°F = 180°C
400°F = 205°C
450°F = 230°C

Weight (Mass) Measurements

1 ounce = 30 grams
2 ounces = 55 grams
3 ounces = 85 grams
4 ounces = ¼ pound = 125 grams
8 ounces = ½ pound = 240 grams
12 ounces = ¾ pound = 375 grams
16 ounces = 1 pound = 454 grams